Challenges and Opportunities for Precision and Personalized Nutrition

PROCEEDINGS OF A WORKSHOP

Emily A. Callahan, *Rapporteur*

Food Forum

Food and Nutrition Board

Health and Medicine Division

The National Academies of
SCIENCES · ENGINEERING · MEDICINE

THE NATIONAL ACADEMIES PRESS
Washington, DC
www.nap.edu

THE NATIONAL ACADEMIES PRESS   500 Fifth Street, NW   Washington, DC 20001

This activity was supported by contracts between the National Academy of Sciences and the National Institutes of Health (HHSN263201800029I/HHSN26300023); the U.S. Department of Agriculture (59-8040-0-001 and 123A9420P0008); and the U.S. Food and Drug Administration (75F40120C00192), with additional support from Academy of Nutrition and Dietetics; American Heart Association; American Institute for Cancer Research; American Society for Nutrition; Cargill, Inc.; Coca-Cola Company; Conagra Brands; Center for Science in the Public Interest; Danone North America; General Mills, Inc.; Keurig Dr Pepper; Mars, Inc.; Mondelēz International; Ocean Spray Cranberries, Inc.; and Unilever. Any opinions, findings, conclusions, or recommendations expressed in this publication do not necessarily reflect the views of any organization or agency that provided support for the project.

International Standard Book Number-13: 978-0-309-08735-3
International Standard Book Number-10: 0-309-08735-X
Digital Object Identifier: https://doi.org/10.17226/26299

Additional copies of this publication are available for sale from the National Academies Press, 500 Fifth Street, NW, Keck 360, Washington, DC 20001; (800) 624-6242 or (202) 334-3313; http://www.nap.edu.

Suggested citation: National Academies of Sciences, Engineering, and Medicine. 2022. *Challenges and opportunities for precision and personalized nutrition: Proceedings of a workshop*. Washington, DC: The National Academies Press. https://doi.org/10.17226/26299.

PLANNING COMMITTEE FOR A WORKSHOP ON CHALLENGES AND OPPORTUNITIES FOR PRECISION AND PERSONALIZED NUTRITION[1]

ERIC A. DECKER (*Chair*), Professor and Head, Department of Food Science, University of Massachusetts Amherst

CINDY DAVIS, National Program Leader for Human Nutrition, Agricultural Research Service, U.S. Department of Agriculture

KATIE KOECHER, Associate Expert Nutrition Scientist, Bell Institute of Health and Nutrition, General Mills, Inc.

BRUCE Y. LEE, Professor and Executive Director, Public Health, Public Health Computational and Operations Research Center for Advanced Technology in Communications and Health, City University of New York School of Public Health & Health Policy

JOSIEMER MATTEI, Donald and Sue Pritzker Associate Professor of Nutrition, Harvard T.H. Chan School of Public Health

ROBIN McKINNON, Senior Advisor for Nutrition Policy, Center for Food Safety and Applied Nutrition, U.S. Food and Drug Administration

NICHOLAS J. SCHORK, Deputy Director and Distinguished Professor, Translational Genomics Research Institute

PATRICK J. STOVER, Vice Chancellor and Dean, Agriculture and Life Sciences, Director, Texas A&M University, Texas A&M AgriLife Research

STEVEN ZEISEL, Professor of Nutrition and Pediatrics, University of North Carolina at Chapel Hill and UNC Nutrition Research Institute, Founder and Board Member, SNP Therapeutics

---

[1] The National Academies of Sciences, Engineering, and Medicine's planning committees are solely responsible for organizing the workshop, identifying topics, and choosing speakers. The responsibility for the published Proceedings of a Workshop rests with the workshop rapporteur and the institution.

v

MEGAN NECHANICKY, General Mills, Golden Valley, Minnesota
RONI NEFF, The Johns Hopkins University, Baltimore, Maryland
SARAH OHLHORST, American Society for Nutrition, Rockville, Maryland
GITA RAMPERSAD, Feeding America, Washington, DC
JILL REEDY, Division of Cancer Prevention, National Cancer Institute, National Institutes of Health, Bethesda, Maryland
KRISTIN REIMERS, Conagra Brands, Omaha, Nebraska
BRIAN RONHOLM, Consumer Reports, Washington, DC
SHARON A. ROSS, Division of Cancer Prevention, National Cancer Institute, National Institutes of Health, Bethesda, Maryland
KELSEY FREEMAN SAELENS, Cargill, Inc., Washington, DC
PAMELA STARKE-REED, Agricultural Research Service, U.S. Department of Agriculture, Beltsville, Maryland
ALISON L. STEIBER, Academy of Nutrition and Dietetics, Chicago, Illinois
MARY T. STORY, Duke University, Durham, North Carolina
PATRICK J. STOVER, Texas A&M University, College Station
CHERYL TONER, American Heart Association, Washington, DC
DOROTHEA K. VAFIADIS, National Council on Aging, Arlington, Virginia

Health and Medicine Division Staff

HEATHER DEL VALLE COOK, Director, Food Forum
CYPRESS LYNX, Research Associate
MARIAH BRUNS, Senior Program Assistant (as of January 2022)
ANN L. YAKTINE, Director, Food and Nutrition Board

Reviewers

This Proceedings of a Workshop was reviewed in draft form by individuals chosen for their diverse perspectives and technical expertise. The purpose of this independent review is to provide candid and critical comments that will assist the National Academies of Sciences, Engineering, and Medicine in making each published proceedings as sound as possible and to ensure that it meets the institutional standards for quality, objectivity, evidence, and responsiveness to the charge. The review comments and draft manuscript remain confidential to protect the integrity of the process. We thank the following individuals for their review of this proceedings:

ERIC A. DECKER, University of Massachusetts Amherst
KATIE KOECHER, General Mills, Inc.
JOSIEMER MATTEI, Harvard T.H. Chan School of Public Health
ROBIN McKINNON, U.S. Food and Drug Administration

Although the reviewers listed above provided many constructive comments and suggestions, they were not asked to endorse the content of the proceedings, nor did they see the final draft before its release. The review of this proceedings was overseen by **JOHANNA T. DWYER,** Tufts Medical Center. She was responsible for making certain that an independent examination of this proceedings was carried out in accordance with standards of the National Academies and that all review comments were carefully considered. Responsibility for the final content rests entirely with the rapporteur and the National Academies.

Contents

Box and Figures

1

Introduction

A virtual workshop titled Challenges and Opportunities for Precision and Personalized Nutrition, held August 10–12, 2021, was convened by the Food Forum of the National Academies of Sciences, Engineering, and Medicine.[1] Planning committee chair Eric A. Decker, University of Massachusetts Amherst, welcomed participants and provided a brief overview of the Food Forum and the workshop. The workshop's objective was to explore potential challenges and opportunities in the application of precision and personalized nutrition approaches to optimize dietary guidance and improve nutritional status.

The workshop opened with a review of the current evidence base, including potential definitions for precision and personalized nutrition, research designs and methodologies, and limitations in design and data (Chapter 2). The session that followed explored innovative methodologies and technologies at the genetic, physiologic/microbiome, individual, and social-ecologic scales of precision nutrition (Chapter 3). The final session addressed implementation of precision and personalized nutrition, including academic, regulatory, and industry perspectives on opportunities and challenges (Chapter 4). The workshop agenda, acronyms and abbreviations used in this publication, and biographical sketches of the workshop

---

[1] The workshop agenda, presentations, and other materials are available at https://www.nationalacademies.org/event/08-10-2021/challenges-and-opportunities-for-precision-and-personalized-nutrition-a-workshop (accessed October 15, 2021).

speakers and planning committee members can be found in Appendixes A, B, and C, respectively. The workshop's statement of task is presented in Box 1-1.[2]

BOX 1-1
Workshop Statement of Task

A planning committee of the National Academies of Sciences, Engineering, and Medicine will plan and convene a public workshop that will explore potential challenges and opportunities in the application of precision and personalized nutrition approaches to optimize dietary guidance and improve nutritional status. Broadly, the workshop sessions will include discussions about the state of the evidence on precision and personalized nutrition, including research gaps, implementation science, and policy challenges.

Workshop presenters will discuss ways to define precision and personalized nutrition and describe how different sources of individual variability (such as genetics, food behavior, and environmental exposures) may affect these definitions and responses to a precision nutrition approach. Workshop presentations may also include topics such as limitations and opportunities for current and new research methodologies, innovations and challenges in the public and private sector, implications for food science, equitable access to precision and personalized nutrition, and the potential impact of these approaches on future dietary guidance. Case studies may be presented to illustrate applications of new research methodologies and precision and personalized nutrition in clinical settings.

---

[2] The workshop planning committee's role was limited to planning the workshop. This Proceedings of a Workshop was prepared by an independent rapporteur as a factual summary of what occurred at the workshop. Statements, recommendations, and opinions expressed are those of independent presenters and participants, and are not necessarily endorsed or verified by the National Academies of Sciences, Engineering, and Medicine, nor should they be construed as reflecting any group consensus.

2

The Current Evidence Base
and Limitations

The August 10 session of the workshop featured six presentations reviewing the current evidence base for precision and personalized nutrition, including potential definitions for these terms, research designs and methodologies, limitations in designs and data, and future challenges and opportunities for the field. Cindy Davis, Agricultural Research Service, U.S. Department of Agriculture, moderated the speaker presentations and an ensuing panel discussion.

HUMAN VARIABILITY: A BASIS FOR PRECISION AND PERSONALIZED NUTRITION

John Mathers, Newcastle University (United Kingdom), discussed human variability and how it serves as a basis for developing precision and personalized nutrition. He began by observing that people differ from each other in visible ways, such as height and body shape, as well as in ways that are less apparent, such as responses to specific foods and diets. To illustrate the latter, Mathers referenced two examples of people exhibiting different responses to the same nutrition intervention. The DIETFITS (Diet Intervention Examining the Factors Interacting with Treatment Success) study, which enrolled more than 600 adults in a 12-month weight loss trial, assessed changes in weight resulting from either a low-fat or a low-carbohydrate diet. In both diet groups, he reported, individual weight loss at the 12-month mark ranged from 25 or more kilograms to no loss, and some participants had even gained weight (up to 10 kilograms) (Gardner et al., 2018). He noted that interindividual differences have also been observed in response to supplemental fish oil, a substance expected to lower the blood concentration of triacylglycerol: Among more than 300 people taking fish oil supplements, some experienced such decreases, but a considerable proportion did not and were deemed "nonresponders" (Madden et al., 2011).

Mathers moved on to discuss interindividual differences in glycemic responses to eating, which he identified as a useful way to begin exploring variation in individuals' metabolic responses to foods. He stated that continuous monitoring of blood glucose concentration to estimate glycemic responses to food is easy and poses a low burden for participants, adding that differences in responses may be related to health outcomes. He highlighted a study in which changes in participants' postmeal blood glucose concentrations were monitored continuously for 1 week, and large interindividual variation was observed in glycemic responses to several types of standardized meals (Zeevi et al., 2015).

Mathers raised the issue of how information on interindividual variation in responses to diet might be applied to the public health challenge of improving population-wide eating habits. Current public health approaches to changing diet are relatively ineffective, he contended, as they typically consist of similar advice for everyone (e.g., eat more fruits and vegetables). He speculated whether a precision or personalized nutrition approach, in which the individual is placed at the center, might lead to nutrition advice and support that would be more effective at improving population health relative to "one-size-fits-all" guidance.

Mathers shared proposed definitions for personalized nutrition and precision nutrition. He defined personalized nutrition as an approach that uses information on individual characteristics to develop targeted nutritional advice, products, or services. Precision nutrition, on the other hand, suggests the possibility of obtaining a sufficient quantitative understanding of the complex relationships among an individual, their food consumption, and their phenotype (including health) to offer nutritional intervention or advice that is known to be individually beneficial. Precision nutrition is more ambitious, Mathers clarified, as it demands much greater scientific certainty (Ordovas et al., 2018).

These definitions raise questions, Mathers continued, about the biological basis for interindividual variation and whether knowledge of that biological basis could be used to develop more effective personalized or precision nutrition. He outlined relevant biological features that influence an individual's responses to food and ultimately long-term health—genotype, the epigenome,[1] and the gut microbiome—and suggested that complex relationships exist between those features and psychological factors.

---

[1] The collection of genetic marks on DNA within a single cell that instruct the genome (NHGRI, 2020).

As an example, Mathers recounted a study in which participants underwent the same measurements on two occasions. First, they consumed a test meal while researchers assessed their satiety responses using an objective biological measure and a subjective, self-reported measure. Participants were then informed that they had either a high-risk or protective genotype for the development of obesity, based on random assignment (not their actual genotype). One week later, the same measurements were repeated following the same test meal. Among individuals who had been told that they had the high-risk gene, no differences were reported in satiety responses measured objectively or subjectively between the two test meals. In contrast, Mathers continued, individuals who had been told that they had the protective gene exhibited substantial increases in both objective and subjective measures of satiety (Turnwald et al., 2019). According to Mathers, these results suggest that learning one's genetic risk changes physiology independently of actual genetic risk, a finding that, if replicated, has implications for using genetic information in the design of precision or personalized nutrition interventions.

Mathers appealed for consideration of a biopsychosocial model—which encompasses biological, psychosocial, and social factors that contribute to interindividual variation—when developing precision and personalized nutrition approaches. He explained that the way these different types of factors affect an individual's response to diet depends on the time scale. For example, glycemic responses to eating manifest during the first 2–3 hours postmeal, with almost all interindividual variation in responses resulting from biological factors. Responses that manifest over longer periods of time (e.g., months, years), such as insulin resistance or development of diabetes, he pointed out, are likely influenced at least equally, if not more so, by psychological and social factors that drive eating behaviors.

Mathers proposed that differences in people's health aspirations, general likes and dislikes, and food preferences are examples of factors to be considered when attempting to change eating behaviors using precision or personalized nutrition approaches. He also suggested that such approaches need to identify and account for barriers to and facilitators of dietary change for an individual.

Next, Mathers discussed inequity in diet and health. In the United Kingdom, he reported, the prevalence of obesity in children at ages 4 and 10 years is twice as high among those from the most deprived compared with the least deprived families. Prevalence increases steadily in both age groups, he added, as the level of deprivation[2] increases (NHS Digital, 2014). As another example, he pointed to data showing that in the United States,

---

[2] Based on the English Indices of Deprivation, available here: https://assets.publishing. service.gov.uk/government/uploads/system/uploads/attachment_data/file/6871/1871208.pdf (accessed October 11, 2021).

life expectancy has increased at the population level over the past several decades, but has done so to a lesser extent among the lowest-income individuals since 2000, an inequity that he stated is linked to socioeconomic differences (Chetty et al., 2016). Mathers asserted that the goal is to develop precision and personalized nutrition approaches that address inequities in dietary intake and health outcomes by improving opportunities for everyone.

Mathers then outlined challenges for precision and personalized nutrition at the individual and societal levels. For individuals, he emphasized the importance of making such approaches accessible, attractive, and acceptable so they create new, motivating opportunities to improve health. At the societal level, he argued for greater reach, affordability, and cost-effectiveness of precision and personalized nutrition approaches, as well as structures that sustain long-term behavior changes.

In closing, Mathers stated that personalized nutrition approaches have been shown to improve adults' dietary intake (Celis-Morales et al., 2017; Jinnette et al., 2021). He suggested that the effectiveness of these approaches could be improved by taking a systems approach. Such an approach, he said, would link information on an individual's characteristics (including barriers to and facilitators of change and aspirations) to a specific self-monitoring process that would feed back to those characteristics in a continuous cycle toward improved health.

PRECISION NUTRITION AT THE INTERSECTION OF HISTORY AND GENOMICS

Constance Hilliard, University of North Texas, began by pointing out that the genetic data on which precision approaches to health are based are often derived from people of European ancestry. The effectiveness of those approaches for improving health in other populations is thereby hindered, she maintained. She then elaborated on the need for precision in dealing with genetic populations by sharing a case study of the etiology of high rates of hypertension and kidney failure in African Americans of slave descent.

Hilliard observed that medical researchers have long searched for explanations for the high prevalence of salt-sensitive hypertension in this segment of the population, which she described as a "crisis situation" based on its linkage to kidney failure, cardiovascular disease, and other comorbidities. Research with inhabitants of West African coastal cities did not replicate the same high rates of hypertension observed in African Americans of slave descent, she recounted, suggesting that a key problem in explaining the latter phenomenon is the medical community's lack of precise knowledge of the ecological niche from which these African Americans originated.

To fill that knowledge gap, Hilliard stated, it is necessary to address three fallacies related to the origins of this population. First, she explained, race is not a scientific concept, and is not suitable for use in medicine except for purposes related to addressing discrimination and past exclusion. Second, DNA ancestry provides a much sharper focus for medical research, she maintained, and understanding ecological niche populations further enhances precision. Third, she pointed out that many ancestors of Black Americans emanated from the deep interior of West Africa, and ended up on the coast only after having been kidnapped and marched up to 1,000 miles to reach waiting slave ships. This detail is critical, she stressed, because coastal West Africans and Europeans were genetically accustomed to consuming 5,000 mg/day of sodium, whereas subsistence farmers in the interior—one of the most sodium-deficient regions in the world—had become genetically adapted to diets providing only 200 mg/day. These farmers were in the lowest echelons of that society, Hilliard added, making them vulnerable to being kidnapped by slave traders.

Hilliard highlighted advances in genomics and genetics leading to the identification of two genetic variants that play a major role in sodium metabolism and are found almost exclusively in people whose ancestors originated in the West African interior. She reported that the presence of either of these variants has been associated with a 2- to 100-fold increased risk of developing kidney disease (NIH, 2017).

Hilliard went on to observe that, based on average sodium intakes of about 3,400 mg/day in the United States (USDA, 2020), African Americans of slave descent consume about 1,700 percent more sodium compared with their ancestors who had adapted to the low-sodium interior region of West Africa, whereas Americans of European ancestry and recent West African immigrants to the United States consume about 32 percent less sodium compared with their ancestors. To improve the health of two diverse genetic populations, then, Hilliard called for stratifying approaches not by race but by DNA ancestry and ecological niche.

On that note, Hilliard turned to a theoretical model of ancestral gene variants that she developed to illustrate that African Americans are admixed populations—for example, 75 percent Niger-Kordofanian West African and 25 percent northern European. This model, she elaborated, suggests that multiplying an individual's percentage of genetic ancestry by the daily sodium consumption levels in healthy members of that population group and then adding the products yields an appropriate average daily sodium intake for the admixed individual. She explained that this model was translated into a theoretical equation (Figure 2-1) that can be used to calculate critical nutrient values in any ecological niche population (where $C_{admixed}$ is the healthy nutrient intake for each segment of admixed ancestry):

$$C_{admixed} = \sum_{i=1}^{n} prop_i \times C_i$$

FIGURE 2-1 The Hilliard-Wang ancestral gene variants theoretical equation for critical nutrient values in any ecological niche population.
SOURCE: Presented by Constance Hilliard on August 10, 2021.

According to Hilliard, the key takeaway is that 21st-century nutrition and health research continues to operate according to a "one-size-fits-all paradigm" that she characterized as outdated, yet powerful because it is invisible and unexamined. The *Dietary Guidelines for Americans* advises those aged 14 years and older to consume less than 2,300 mg/day of sodium, she pointed out, but this is substantially higher than the amounts consumed by the ancestors of African Americans of slave descent (USDA and HHS, 2020).

To conclude her presentation, Hilliard maintained that modern genomics and testing of DNA ancestry provide the opportunity to bring greater precision to sodium guidelines and other nutrient guidance for all Americans. From her perspective, these tools introduce the possibility of stratifying nutrition guidance by DNA ancestry instead of providing standardized guidance that she suggested disadvantages certain populations. Certain disease triggers vary from one genetic population to another, she stressed, and data available to provide precise guidance for one genetic population may be meaningless for other genetic populations. The idea of stratifying guidance implies the need to view Americans as not only multiethnic or multiracial, she argued, but also multigenomic.

INTEGRATING MICROBIOME AND DIETARY DATA

Abigail Johnson, University of Minnesota, discussed potential approaches for integrating information about the microbiome with data on dietary intake. She began by explaining that dramatic shifts in microbiome development and composition occur from infancy through early toddlerhood, corresponding with such dietary changes as initiation of breastfeeding or formula feeding and introduction of complementary foods. Microbiome composition reaches a more stable point by adulthood, she said, with some variation that can be attributed to seasonality, geographic location, movement between countries, exposure to antibiotics, and medical events, for example.

It is becoming increasingly apparent, Johnson emphasized, that the microbiome is shaped by the foods a person eats and is also an independent contributor to that person's diet-related health outcomes. She explained that nutrition scientists and researchers have long understood that dietary intake, with some variation from genetics, influences the phenotypes expressed and often is associated with health or disease conditions, but that the picture is clearer when the microbiome's contribution is included. As an example, she pointed out that the microbiome modifies and produces dietary metabolites that were not previously considered but may have a role in the development of health outcomes (Figure 2-2).

Johnson described her postdoctoral research study, whose objective was to characterize day-to-day changes in the composition of the adult microbiome resulting from dietary intake. She explained that 34 study participants collected one microbiome (stool) sample daily for 17 days, and her research team analyzed the composition of each participant's samples. One type of analysis reduced the complexity of the multiple species in each participant's microbiome to two or three principal components, which captured the greatest possible variation among the microbiomes. In this type of analysis, each participant's microbiome conformation was plotted as a single point on a coordinate plane. The farther apart the points, Johnson explained, the more distinct and different from each other were the microbiomes represented by the points, whereas overlapping points would indicate microbiomes that were essentially identical. This analysis revealed that participants had distinct microbiome conformations, she recounted, and that those conformations were relatively unchanged from day to day.

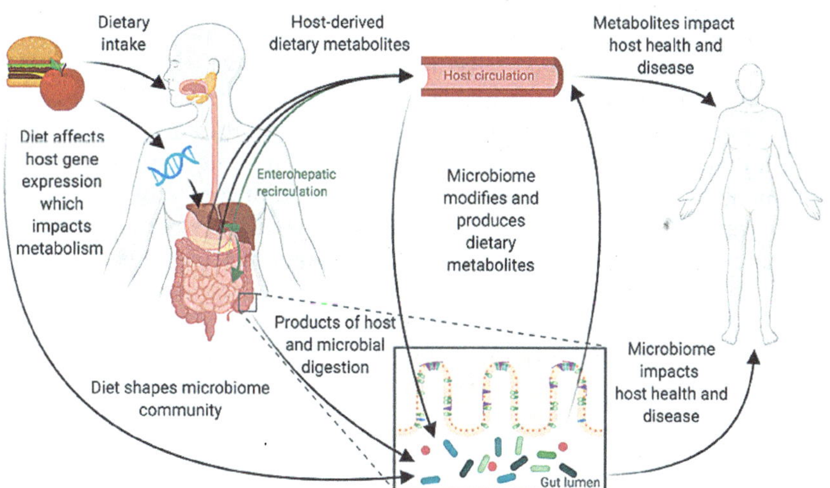

FIGURE 2-2 The microbiome is a product of diet and an influence on diet-related health outcomes.
SOURCES: Presented by Abigail Johnson on August 10, 2021; Johnson et al., 2020. Reprinted with permission from *Frontiers in Nutrition*.

The best way to integrate dietary and microbiome data was not immediately clear, Johnson acknowledged, and her team chose to collect participants' dietary records for the 24 hours prior to each of the 17 daily microbiome samples. The researchers analyzed the dietary records in a way that enabled them to visualize the relative abundance of different food groups, which Johnson said made clear that dietary composition was more variable than corresponding microbiome composition from day to day. Dietary data were also analyzed using network visualization, a computational tool commonly used in microbiome research, to illustrate the number of people who ate each food reported in the dietary records. This visualization showed that some foods were consumed by many participants and others by only one or two. Another level of analysis determined the macronutrient and micronutrient composition of foods consumed by study participants, Johnson reported, confirming that nutrient intake was more stable than individual food intake during the study period. She described another computational tool common in microbiome research, Procrustes analysis, which was applied to assess how dietary intake influenced microbiome composition and showed that the participants' microbiomes did not pair with the nutrients they consumed.

At this point, Johnson recounted, the team reconsidered its approach to assessing food intake, and the concept of "dietary dark matter" came to the fore. She described this as the myriad of biochemicals, such as polyphenols, flavors, and other compounds, that are present in a given food—many in minute amounts—and serve as substrates for bacteria, but are rarely quantified or studied to the same extent as essential nutrients. She pointed out that even small particles of food arrive in the lumen relatively intact even after digestion has occurred in the higher gastrointestinal tract, which suggests that they could have an impact on different communities of gut bacteria.

On that note, Johnson turned to discussing an additional approach to examining dietary intake. This approach, she said, incorporates the highly multivariate nature dietary of intake similarly to what has been done in microbiome analyses. Microbiome data can be organized in terms of specific species, she explained, and amounts of those species present in a sample can be quantified. Her team applied this approach to dietary intake by clustering the foods consumed into food groups and generating a phenetic tree to account statistically for similarities among foods with respect to their food group characteristics (Figure 2-3). It thereby became possible to apply additional tools from the microbiome space to explore diet, such as UniFrac, a distance metric used for comparing biological communities. Applied to dietary data, Johnson reported, UniFrac distance generated multivariate ordinations that revealed the distinct and highly variable nature of each study participant's dietary patterns. When Procrustes analysis was applied to average microbiome composition and average food composition in the

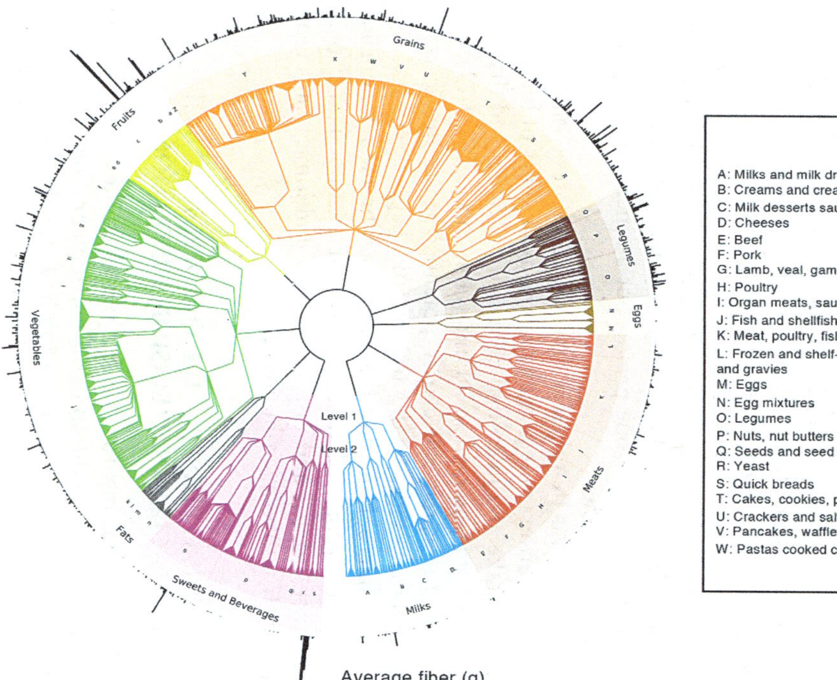

FIGURE 2-3 A phenetic tree for use in accounting for food groups and their relatedness.
SOURCES: Presented by Abigail Johnson on August 10, 2021; Johnson et al., 2019. Reprinted with permission from Elsevier.

ordination generated by the UniFrac distance method, microbiome composition successfully paired with food intake. Both grain fiber diversity and fruit fiber diversity (a metric based on the diversity of fiber from grains and fruit instead of the overall quantity of those food groups) also paired with microbiome composition using this method.

According to Johnson, the ordination resulting from the UniFrac distance method also led the research team to determine that dietary patterns driven by consumption of alcohols, fats, poultry, grains, and cakes (i.e., similar to Western, high-fat diets) appeared to be associated with the abundance of specific bacterial species. Further analysis indicated that these dietary patterns explained a large amount of the variation in the microbiome and revealed a *Bacteroidetes* gradient.

Turning to the application of these findings to precision and personalized nutrition approaches, Johnson reported that the method applying UniFrac distance and Procrustes analysis identified significant agreement between diet and microbiome for 28 of the 34 study participants when the respective 17 days of data were considered longitudinally for each individual. Moreover, she continued, the research team found that most diet–microbe associations were personalized—i.e., a large number of significant relationships existed between foods and bacterial species within a person, but few of those relationships were repeated across people. For example, consumption of dark green vegetables was correlated with a decrease in a specific *Bacteroidetes* species in one person but an increase in the same *Bacteroidetes* species in another.

Johnson's final point was that dietary diversity correlates with microbiome stability, an observation made possible by the availability of longitudinal data on dietary intake and microbial composition. She noted that this relationship has also been observed in infants (Homann et al., 2021), and suggested that further research will clarify potential health implications. Finally, she reiterated that foods and dietary patterns shape the composition and dynamics of the microbiome and that diet–microbiome relationships are individualized, and proposed that multivariate dietary data can be thought of as another "-ome" and integrated with multiomics data using computational tools from the microbiome space.

AN ENGINEERING PERSPECTIVE ON OPPORTUNITIES AND OBSTACLES IN PRECISION NUTRITION

Christian Metallo, Salk Institute for Biological Studies, discussed the application of metabolomics to the study of nutrition and disease physiology, illustrated by a case study demonstrating how metabolic mechanisms affect the balance of nonessential amino acids and drive a particular disease state.

Precision and personalized nutrition can absolutely be used to modulate health, Metallo asserted, but he maintained that more sophisticated understanding of the body's robust, genetic biochemical engineering control mechanisms (i.e., metabolism) is needed to exploit those mechanisms therapeutically through diet. Static metabolite measurements have limited utility, he added, but can be enhanced with information about the location and dynamics of the processes by which the metabolites are derived.

Metallo presented a case study of macular telangiectasia (MacTel)—a disease of the macula, the part of the eye that is responsible for high visual resolution and accounts for about half of neural activity in the retina. MacTel is characterized by vascular abnormalities that are observed by fluorescein angiogram, he explained, and manifests in central vision loss and difficulties with such activities as driving and reading at a relatively young age (~40 years) in affected individuals. He noted that MacTel is a familial disease with a large genetic component, and an international group of scientists and clinicians was convened in 2005 to better understand its causes.

Since then, Metallo continued, genome-wide association studies (GWAS) have identified several specific genetic variations in MacTel patients that are associated with the serine (a nonessential amino acid) biosynthesis pathway, such that serine and glycine levels are lower in the plasma of MacTel patients compared with controls. Serine and glycine are involved in a number of metabolic pathways, he said, and give rise to numerous downstream metabolites.

Metallo's team sought to understand serine's role in the development of MacTel by examining how cells control flux of a substrate (serine) to different pathways. Because numerous enzymes compete for serine in cells, Metallo explained, evolution has attuned the most important enzymes to have a high affinity for serine so they can bind it when concentrations are low. The team identified serine palmitoyl transferase (SPT) as a key enzyme and recognized that it normally uses serine to catalyze biosynthesis of sphingolipids (structural components of cell membranes), but can also use alanine to generate deoxysphingolipids if serine levels are low or if specific mutations are present in subunits of SPT. MacTel patients have higher levels of deoxysphingolipids relative to control patients, Metallo noted, and plasma levels of the metabolite 1-deoxysphinganine are also increased in patients with another type of hereditary neuropathy (some but not all of whom have MacTel) that is responsible for peripheral neuropathy and loss of thermal sensing.

Metallo's team next examined whether dietary manipulation could drive a neurological phenotype similar to that observed in MacTel patients. They fed mice a serine/glycine-free diet and observed that after 10 months, the mice had lost thermal sensing and were exhibiting some retinal defect. The team concluded that the same phenotype as that driven by genetics in MacTel patients could also be caused by an atypical diet.

Metallo reported that several lines of genetic evidence are now available to clarify that MacTel is a multigenic disease of dysregulated amino acid metabolism, characterized by a metabolic phenotype in which levels of serine and glycine are low and levels of alanine are elevated. This discovery, he observed, has prompted additional questions about whether other factors, dietary or otherwise, influence this phenotype, and whether the phenotype is linked to more common diseases and comorbidities, such as type 2 diabetes. Metallo's team explored this question by attempting to accelerate peripheral neuropathy via additional dietary manipulations. They found that a metabolic imbalance was triggered with a serine- and glycine-free low-fat diet, as well as with a serine- and glycine-adequate high-fat diet, but the combination of a serine- and glycine-free and Western-style high-fat (60 percent of energy intake from fat) diet triggered the "metabolic catastrophe" that led to peripheral neuropathy. This is a severe and extreme diet, Metallo admitted, raising questions about how the metabolic pathway leading to peripheral neuropathy might function in individuals consuming a more typical diet.

Metallo then turned to another research question arising from the case study: whether there is a way to identify type 2 diabetes patients who are susceptible to peripheral neuropathy. This question arose, he explained, because it appears that metabolic syndrome steers metabolism in such a way as to reduce serine levels and cause peripheral neuropathy associated with serine deficiency in some patients. Specifically, the research team wondered whether they could identify an assay that could be used to confirm whether a person with diabetes is experiencing serine deficiency, similar to the way in which a glucose tolerance test reveals insulin resistance. A serine tolerance test could enable more direct quantification of serine/glycine disposal, he suggested, which is an indicator of whether serine supplementation may be an effective therapy for a particular patient with diabetes.

PSYCHOSOCIAL INFLUENCES ON EATING BEHAVIOR

Susan Carnell, Johns Hopkins University School of Medicine, discussed how psychosocial and behavioral research on eating behavior can enhance precision nutrition not only by determining an optimal diet for an individual but also by identifying the best strategies for supporting that individual in following the diet. To lay a foundation for her presentation, she referred to a biopsychosocial model of factors that influence the development of obesity (Figure 2-4) and highlighted eating behaviors in its psychological compartment.

Carnell began by defining the term "appetitive characteristics" as early-emerging, enduring dispositions toward food or eating styles that differ among individuals. As examples of appetitive characteristics, she cited food cue responsiveness (the degree to which a person responds to external

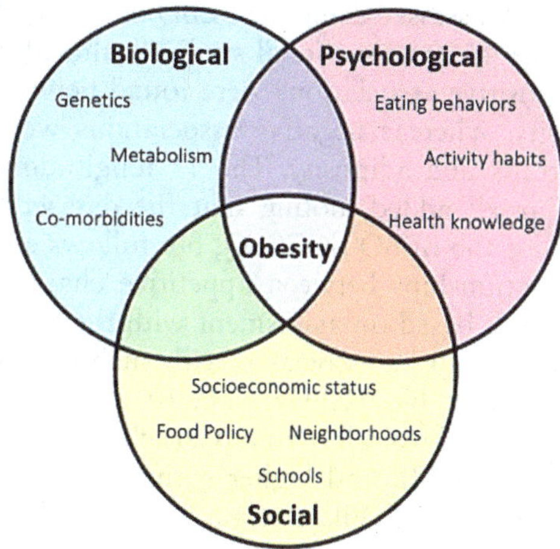

FIGURE 2-4 The biopsychosocial model as it relates to the development of obesity.
SOURCE: Presented by Susan Carnell on August 10, 2021.

food cues, such as the sight or smell of food) and satiety responsiveness (a person's level of sensitivity to internal cues to stop eating, such as gut hormones or gastric distension) (Carnell and Wardle, 2008).

Appetitive characteristics can be measured with behavioral tests or questionnaires, Carnell continued, noting that the latter might be more useful for developing personalized nutrition plans for children. She described an instrument commonly used with children—the Child Eating Behavior Questionnaire (CEBQ), a parental-report measure of a child's traits associated with food approach (e.g., food responsiveness, enjoyment of food, and emotional overeating) or food avoidance (e.g., satiety responsiveness, slowness in eating, food fussiness, and emotional undereating) (Wardle et al., 2001). She added that a version of the questionnaire for infants—the Baby Eating Behavior Questionnaire (BEBQ)—assesses the same traits during the period in which a child consumes only breastmilk and/or infant formula (Llewellyn et al., 2011), and that a version for adults (AEBQ) was developed more recently (Hunot et al., 2016). With regard to the population prevalence of the traits measured by these questionnaires, Carnell shared unpublished data from a community survey of several hundred children (aged 2–12 years) and adults, indicating lower satiety responsiveness and higher food responsiveness and emotional overeating among adults compared with children.

Carnell next discussed relationships between appetitive characteristics and weight/adiposity. She started by highlighting a systematic review and meta-analysis of data on more than 36,000 children aged 1–14 years whose eating behaviors were assessed using the BEBQ or CEBQ (Kininmoth et al., 2020). Based on the 46 cross-sectional studies included in the review, she reported, robust positive associations were found between food approach traits and adiposity, whereas negative associations were found between food avoidance traits and adiposity. The 11 longitudinal studies yielded similar results, Carnell added, noting that the dataset for the AEBQ is smaller than that for the BEBQ or CEBQ, but follows a similar pattern.

Moving to relationships between appetitive characteristics and diet, Carnell reported that, based on assessment with the CEBQ, higher satiety responsiveness appears to be associated with such outcomes as lower affinity for fruits and vegetables (Fildes et al., 2015), less fruit and vegetable intake as a percentage of overall intake (Carnell et al., 2016), less dietary variety (Vilela et al., 2018), and higher eating frequencies (i.e., perhaps more of a snacking pattern) (Vilela et al., 2019). Preliminary analyses of AEBQ data from Carnell's recent community survey support similar patterns in adults, but to date are unpublished. According to Carnell, these findings indicate that both appetite and food preferences/habits are important considerations for developing personalized nutrition approaches.

Turning to the influence of genetics on eating behavior, Carnell presented data from a study that assessed satiety responsiveness and food enjoyment in pairs of twins aged 8–11 years. Correlations for both traits were much higher among monozygotic twins (those who share all of their genes) than dizygotic twins (those who share half their genes), with heritability calculations attributing 63 percent of the variation in satiety responsiveness and 75 percent of the variation in enjoyment of food to genetics. Carnell remarked further that traits of emotional overeating and undereating showed more environmental than genetic influence. She reported that data on heritability of appetitive characteristics among infants indicate that slowness in eating and satiety responsiveness are substantially influenced by genetics, as are enjoyment of food and food responsiveness (Llewellyn et al., 2010). According to Carnell, an implication of these findings is that because appetitive behaviors appear to emerge early in life and are genetically determined to some extent, it may be better to work with them than against them as they may be difficult to change (Carnell et al., 2008).

Carnell next discussed binge eating as another example of eating behavior, with some individuals meeting criteria for binge eating disorder as defined in the *Diagnostic and Statistical Manual of Mental Disorders, Fifth Edition* (DSM-5). According to that definition, binge eating disorder is characterized by recurrent (at least once per week) and persistent (≥ 3 months) binge eating episodes in the absence of compensatory behaviors, accompanied by marked distress (Hudson et al., 2007). According to Carnell, its lifetime prevalence in the United States is 2.8 percent. She explained that during an episode of binge eating, a large amount of food is consumed in a short period of time, a behavior often triggered by stress and anxiety and occurring in the evening when an individual is alone. Some individuals may engage in recurrent binge eating episodes without meeting the criteria for binge eating disorder (a behavior termed subthreshold binge eating disorder), she pointed out, and still others may sometimes report subjective experiences of loss of control while eating a reportedly objectively large amount of food (termed binge eating). In adolescents, she added, loss-of-control eating may be present, in which individuals report subjective experiences of loss of control while eating irrespective of the reported amount of food consumed—a behavior reported by about one-third of children and adolescents with overweight or obesity (Tanofsky-Kraff et al., 2020). Carnell noted that the literature describes this type of eating behavior using a variety of terms (e.g., reward-based eating, hedonic eating, food addiction, disinhibited eating) that differ slightly, yet seem to point to an underlying latent trait of uncontrolled eating that is exhibited to varying degrees. Uncontrolled eating, she observed, is related to more general behavioral traits such as reward sensitivity, cognitive control, and negative affect, which she pointed out may all contribute to the expression of uncontrolled eating in an individual and lead to overeating and obesity.

Carnell next discussed the relationships between appetitive characteristics and individual responses to the food environment and to interventions designed to change eating behaviors. Acknowledging that few studies have examined these relationships, she cited one that examined children's responses to variable portion sizes—100, 150, 200, and 250 percent of the recommended amount of food for a meal—and found that children with the highest satiety responsiveness were relatively unaffected by the portion size condition, whereas those with the lowest satiety responsiveness were most likely to increase food intake in response to increasing portion sizes (Mooreville et al., 2015). She also referenced a study of behavioral obesity treatment in which children participated in a family-based weight loss intervention, and children's appetites were found to be associated with their outcomes: children with high satiety responsiveness had positive outcomes (i.e., decreases from baseline in body mass index z-score), even by the 18-month follow-up visit, whereas those with high food responsiveness or high emotional eating had begun regaining weight by the 6-month follow-up visit, suggesting that such children may have more challenges maintaining dietary changes (Boutelle et al., 2019). Finally, Carnell cited an intensive lifestyle intervention targeting weight loss in adults with diabetes, in which the group that displayed consistent binge eating behaviors had lost the least weight at the 4-year mark (Chao et al., 2017). According to Carnell, a key point from these studies is that when designing personalized nutrition plans, it is important to account for eating behaviors that could affect how individuals respond to certain recommendations.

Carnell then commented on the potential influence on eating behaviors of two factors associated with socioeconomic status—food insecurity and stress—and suggested that delay discounting may be involved. Delay discounting is the degree to which an individual is inclined to choose a reward (food or nonfood) that is smaller but delivered sooner as opposed to one that is larger but delivered later. In a study of food-related delay discounting, Carnell reported, women who were food insecure versus those who were food secure were more likely to choose smaller food rewards delivered sooner, suggesting that food insecurity may affect habitual food decisions (Rodriguez et al., 2021). Carnell cited another study, conducted at the beginning of the COVID-19 pandemic, in which psychosocial stress was found to influence the reinforcing value of food—that is, the motivation to obtain or work to obtain food. Motivation to obtain sweet snacks, fruit, and fast foods was greater than motivation to obtain savory snacks and vegetables, she observed, and higher COVID-19-related stress was associated with greater food motivation across all food categories (Smith et al., 2021). Thus, she suggested, psychosocial factors may be another important consideration in the context of personalized nutrition interventions.

Carnell closed by illustrating how eating behaviors could guide personalized nutrition approaches. In terms of eating plans and food environments, for example, someone with low satiety responsiveness might be more successful with portion-controlled meals than with buffet- or family-style meals, and foods with higher satiety value could be emphasized. In contrast, an individual with high satiety responsiveness might tend toward frequent snacking, so guidance for appropriately portioned, nutrient-dense snacks could be useful. If food responsiveness is high, Carnell continued, controlling the dietary environment is important, and those with binge or stress eating patterns might benefit more from maintaining a healthy home food environment to reduce temptation and stressors and to find alternative coping strategies. She suggested that such individuals might also seek treatment involving training in appetite awareness and cue exposure responsiveness (Boutelle et al., 2020).

INTEGRATION OF MULTIPLE OMICS

Michael Snyder, Stanford University, discussed the use of big data to support individualized profiling as a strategy for better managing health. He began by observing that it is increasingly becoming possible to quantify the factors that influence an individual's health, such as one's genome and lifestyle exposures, including stress, diet, physical activity, and environmental pathogens. Importantly, he stressed, the effects of these factors can also be quantified with detailed molecular and physiological measurements of an individual.

Snyder described his group's longitudinal research on personal omics profiling, which involves using in-depth measures to gather information about a person's genome, epigenome, transcriptome, proteome, cytokines, metabolome, lipidome, and microbiome, among others. Questionnaires, basic and advanced clinical tests, and wearable biosensor devices provide additional information, he explained, with the goal of better characterizing what it means to be healthy and describing what a healthy profile looks like, how it changes over time and during phases of illness, and how it differs among individuals. The researchers have followed more than 100 people for about 8 years, he added, taking samples approximately every 3 months while participants are healthy, with additional samples being taken if they become sick or encounter other health challenges. Another objective is to determine whether advanced technologies such as genome sequencing and other deep biological profiling can make a measurable difference in better managing people's health (Schüssler-Fiorenza Rose et al., 2019).

Snyder recounted nearly 50 occurrences of what he called "major health discoveries" during the first 3.5 years of profiling of study participants, including detection of cardiovascular, metabolic, hematological, or oncological abnormalities (such as gene mutations) that often precede disease. Early warning signs were detected by a variety of methods, including wearables, genome sequencing, imaging, and molecular measurements. Snyder noted that no single technology was common to all of the discoveries, but that in many cases, multiple measurements had indicated the anomalies. Importantly, he stressed, every health discovery was made before the affected individual had shown symptoms of the problem, enabling several participants to act early to treat underlying disease.

Snyder's group is also monitoring participants' transitions in status with respect to diabetes, and has observed an increase in the prevalence of diagnosed diabetes and prediabetes among participants over the course of the study. People followed different paths to developing diabetes, Snyder reported, such as weight gain, elevation of fasting blood glucose, or other triggers. This finding has led his group to believe that diabetes (particularly type 2) is a heterogeneous disease and that better understanding of its origins in a given person could lead to better management.

Another lesson learned from the study, Snyder continued, is that people age differently, as revealed by longitudinal molecular measures of various indicators of aging. He listed four general classes of aging molecules—relating to kidney, liver, metabolic, or immune functions and pathways—and suggested that people can be grouped into at least four "ageotypes" based on their rates of change in these pathways. People may age primarily in one category, he explained, or in two, three, or all four categories.

Snyder mentioned a company called Qbio that is scaling up the study's concept of multiple omics profiling, emphasizing the use of longitudinal measurements to detect changes over time and enhance understanding of an individual's health trajectory. Snyder's laboratory is using wearable sensors to collect a large amount of data each day on such biological indicators as heart rate, heart rate variability, respiration, skin temperature, blood oxygen, and blood pressure. Such physiological measures, he explained, can signal the onset of illness in an individual, and his research group was able to develop an algorithm for predicting illness based on changes in resting heart rate data.

Snyder then turned to the considerable potential of wearable devices to aid in rapid detection of illness, such as COVID-19. He gave as an example a smartwatch that can measure physiological events in real time and detect changes presymptomatically, citing it as a tool of interest in a study his group is conducting to examine how changes in heart rate can predict the development of COVID-19. In the latest version of the study, run over the past year, the group used smartwatch and smartphone alerts to notify people of changes in their resting heart rate, which are indicative of stress events, including respiratory viral infections. Snyder reported that the ongoing study successfully identified 80 percent of COVID-positive participants at or prior to symptom onset, and also detected asymptomatic cases. Elevations in heart rate prior to illness can be fairly subtle (e.g., the median difference being an extra 7 beats per minute) but can be detected with continuous measurements.

Snyder went on to point out that smartwatches can collect other clinical biomarkers, such as hemoglobin levels, red blood cell counts, and fasting glucose, which may be no substitute for diagnosis-grade measurements and consultation with a health care provider, but still can provide clues that something may be awry. He referred to a personal health dashboard that can integrate an individual's wearable data and omics and microbiome data on a smartphone interface as they are collected over time, allowing the user to monitor these health measurements as often as desired.

Snyder ended his presentation by describing the example of a study that examined the effects of feeding with different types of dietary fibers. Among the 18 participants, he reported, a drop in low-density lipoprotein (LDL) cholesterol was observed after consumption of both arabinoxylan alone and a combination of arabinoxylan and inulin, but not after consumption of inulin alone. The literature is mixed regarding the effects of each of these fibers on cholesterol, he noted, but is more consistent in explaining the mechanism by which fiber is believed to lower cholesterol (i.e., by binding to it so that it is excreted along with the nondigestible fiber). But in this study, an increase in secondary bile acids was observed with consumption of arabinoxylan, which led researchers to develop a new theory for how that type of fiber lowers cholesterol. Of interest, Snyder observed, in one of the study participants, inulin but not arabinoxylan lowered LDL cholesterol, a finding he said highlights the importance of understanding people at the individual level to better manage their health.

PANEL DISCUSSION

Measures of Contributors to Interindividual Variation

An audience member asked whether it is better to frame interindividual variability as a reflection of the sensitivity of specific biological pathways to bidirectional, complex links to genomic, social, psychological, dietary, and other components instead of framing it in terms of separate biological, psychological, and social domains. According to Snyder, studying various components simultaneously is important because effects are not necessarily linear and can be synergistic. Modeling algorithms have been developed to support multiple inputs in studying nonlinear systems, he pointed out, and results suggest that the effects of individual inputs may differ when presented alone versus in combination with other inputs. According to Mathers, one of the challenges is to measure the variety of nonbiological factors that influence health, for which he suggested that fewer validated, scalable, inexpensive assessment tools exist compared with tools for measuring biological factors.

Interindividual Variation in Effects of Foods on Gut Microbial Species

Johnson proposed that variability among individuals in the effects of specific foods on gut microbial species could be attributed to the failure of dietary intake assessment tools to collect complete information about how a consumed food(s) was prepared. To illustrate this point, she noted that herbs and spices that have been added to a food could influence its effect on gut microbes. She also pointed out that even after controlling for differences in food preparation, variability among individuals in a food's effect on gut microbial species can be attributed to gut microbes cross-feeding and interacting with each other and across kingdoms (i.e., fungal and bacterial cross-feeding networks), rather than acting alone to break down specific foods. Mathers suggested that from the perspective of viewing the gut microbiome as a complex ecosystem where different inhabitants play different roles, it is a "major task" to understand the influences of individual food components. Snyder remarked that more immune cells are present in the gut than anywhere else in the body, indicating that dietary intake is an important influence on immune function.

Communicating Differences in Nutrient Needs by Genetic Population

Asked whether nutrition labels should be changed to reflect variation in nutrient needs, Hilliard emphasized the value of stratifying dietary guidance according to genetic populations, but acknowledged that she was uncertain of the best approach for doing so. She suggested that because of the small number of cases in which one ancestral population has a major genomic difference of consequence for a specific dietary variable, messaging and education might be a better approach than trying to provide multiple different percent daily intake values on a food label, for example, corresponding to different genetic populations. She reiterated that attempts to aggregate data from multiethnic population groups may be framed as diversifying, but contended that diversifying is inferior to stratifying if the goal is to obtain accurate data. Hilliard acknowledged that the diversity of genetic populations represented in the United States makes providing dietary guidance more difficult compared with countries consisting of one or two genetic populations.

Affordability of Individual Profiling Technology

Snyder observed that collecting multiple omics from an individual is expensive—several thousand dollars for the Qbio version—but maintained that its utility for preventing major health outcomes, such as heart attack, is extremely cost-saving, particularly for at-risk groups. He believes that in the future, inexpensive home tests will be available for simple biochemical measurements such as cholesterol and glucose, and reiterated that wearable devices costing as little as $60 each could be distributed at a global level to collect useful health information.

Drivers of Eating Behaviors

Asked whether genes or environments drive eating behaviors, Carnell replied that both are important. Evidence suggests, she said, that food preferences and appetite have genetic components, and also indicates that overconsumption of highly energy-dense foods may down-regulate brain dopamine receptors and cause individuals to be less responsive to those foods, which in turn may actually drive them to seek those foods. Carnell also pointed out that everyone is genetically predisposed to seeking energy-dense foods as a survival mechanism. At the same time, she continued, the availability of such foods also drives their consumption, and food preferences appear to be more influenced by environments than by genetics. Furthermore, she observed, the foods available in a given environment could lead to greater or lesser expression of an individual's genetic propensity for seeking highly energy-dense foods.

Risks of Using Genomic Markers for Early Detection of Disease

Snyder recounted his experience with sequencing genomes of healthy people and making health predictions, noting that he has been cautioned that this activity would lead to millions of dollars in follow-up tests and excessive overdiagnosis (i.e., disease that would not progress to pathology). The actual outcome was not that extreme (rather, a median cost of $700 per person), he recalled, and he contended that follow-up testing and costs are worthwhile when they have the potential to uncover indicators of disease. In terms of the potential for overdiagnosis, Snyder argued that an appropriate perspective on genomic markers of disease is to view them as a screening tool for potential risk factors. He also noted that the individuals involved in his study of multiple omics were enthusiastic participants who indicated that they had derived benefit and not experienced increased stress or anxiety from their participation and knowledge of their omics data.

Scalability of Metabolomics to Examine Disease Pathology

Metallo reminded participants that the MacTel project was made possible by a wealthy donor who was highly motivated to investigate the disease in new ways, but he also pointed out that studying the molecular mechanisms of this single disease led to understanding of different mechanisms that might impact the development of diabetes. He suggested that these kinds of incidental findings may be the most likely way of learning about more diseases via metabolomics because of the challenges of applying a MacTel approach to all major diseases.

Use of Microbiome Measures for Dietary Intake Assessment

Johnson affirmed that dietary intake assessment entails many challenges and predicted that future advances may make it possible to use microbiome data for insight into dietary intake. She referenced other colleagues' efforts to collect data on microbiome responses to single foods and to examine microbial DNA metabarcodes[3] from people on plant- versus animal-based diets to assess the diversity of foods consumed. Mathers suggested that metabolomic data on blood, urine, or saliva, which he said are directly related to individual foods, may be a more readily available tool for dietary assessment.

Effect of Metabolomic Differences on Interindividual Variability

Metallo pointed to the considerable interindividual variation for any given metabolite, which is why his group focused on a specific pathway and tried to examine the dynamics of how metabolite levels fluctuate.

---

[3] Microbial DNA metabarcoding is a method of species identification that uses genetic markers to identify the DNA of a mixture of organisms (Taberlet et al., 2012).

According to Snyder, human data to inform the relationships among food, the microbiome, and metabolites are relatively scarce. Mathers noted that a critical component linking the genome to the metabolome is the Phase 2 enzyme system, which is involved in converting metabolites into urine solutes, the forms of which depend on genetic variation. Therefore, he suggested, understanding of genetic variation will enhance understanding of metabolomics variation. Snyder added that the epigenome is another critical component, referencing the effect of food intake on epigenetic expression, such as DNA methylation.

Biological Mechanisms of Ageotypes

Asked what biological mechanisms can explain the existence of a variety of ageotypes, Snyder responded that the ability to measure different ageotypes is the first step. The second, he continued, is to identify clinical markers associated with different ageotypes, such as hemoglobin A1c for metabolic aging and creatinine for kidney aging, and to learn how such exposures as dietary intake and statin use could affect levels of those markers. According to Hilliard, her research suggests that people digest staple foods from their ancestral diets most efficiently, a finding she believes may have implications for digestive aging when immigrants are brought into new locales where those staple foods are unavailable or less available.

Measuring Personalized Responses in Clinical Trials

Given the limitations of measuring mean response to pharmaceuticals, an audience member asked when the current paradigm of clinical trial design might change to enable personalized responses to be measurable and meaningful for conclusions about efficacy. The landscape is already changing in precision medicine, observed Mathers, where the individual appropriateness of pharmaceuticals is considered. The difficulty, he suggested, is that the current paradigm of clinical trial design has proven effective and is so entrenched in the research community that it is difficult to say when researchers might be willing to change it to address new needs. He predicted that in 10 years, measurement of personalized responses will be more common. Snyder agreed and urged more attention to the concept of distinguishing responders and nonresponders when designing endpoints for clinical trials instead of focusing solely on the average within the study population. Even drugs that have been removed from the market can be highly beneficial for some people, he contended, despite being removed because they were harmful for others. Johnson suggested that clinical trial designs could be enhanced by increasing the density of sampling and the number of time points for data collection. She also cited as a limitation of distinguishing responders from nonresponders the need to define in advance what constitutes a response, as opposed to normal variation that may not be meaningful. In the context of obesity intervention, Carnell pointed to increasing attention to the need to integrate a consistent battery of psychological measures across studies so that individual differences in treatment response can be more fully understood.

Broadening the Accessibility of Precision Nutrition

In response to an audience member's question about recruiting volunteers or attracting customers whose data can help in developing the evidence base for precision nutrition, Johnson observed that precision nutrition technologies are currently being used by the "worried well," and raised the question of how to design approaches that are more widely accessible for people with fewer resources. Hilliard agreed and suggested that wider participation could help identify risk patterns involved in health outcomes for which racial and ethnic disparities exist. Snyder called for government funding, acknowledging that the private sector's efforts are financed by affluent participants. Mathers added that inequity affects whole societies and that as a result, it is important for societies to invest in access to personalized or precision nutrition instead of expecting individuals to self-pay.

Final Thoughts

Davis invited the six speakers to offer final thoughts before concluding the panel discussion. Snyder reiterated the potential value of using multiple omics measurements to inform personalized and precision nutrition approaches to optimizing an individual's health. Hilliard stressed that individuals are members of different genetic populations with variants that have the potential to influence health outcomes. Johnson appealed for making careful, deliberate progress in advancing the field of precision nutrition, instead of rushing to conclusions based on early results. Metallo agreed, and also expressed his excitement about advances that have allowed researchers to examine the molecular origins of disease. Mathers urged stakeholders to ask continually how advances in precision and personalized nutrition will address inequities and improve public health. Finally, Carnell appealed for evaluation of people's psychological and behavioral responses to personal nutrition interventions, with attention to assessment of potential unintended consequences.

3

Innovative Methodologies
and Technologies

The August 11 session of the workshop opened with an overview of the industry landscape in personalized nutrition, which was followed by reviews of selected innovative methodologies and technologies for personalized nutrition at the genetic, physiologic/microbiome, individual, and social-ecologic scales, with each scale being discussed by three speakers. Bruce Y. Lee, City University of New York Graduate School of Public Health & Health Policy, moderated the speaker presentations and an ensuing panel discussion.

INDUSTRY LANDSCAPE IN PERSONALIZED NUTRITION

Mariëtte Abrahams, Qina, reviewed the landscape of the personalized nutrition industry over the past decade. In 2012, she began, limited scientific evidence was available to indicate the impact of giving personalized nutrition advice beyond that in existing medical nutrition therapy guidelines. The market consisted of a few niche players focused on the "worried well," she observed, who could afford personalized guidance. She noted that early adopters tended to be highly educated and affluent females, and the solutions dispensed were based primarily on the data obtained from the specimens of individuals; behavior change was an afterthought that was not incorporated into proposed solutions. Abrahams pointed to a subsequent gradual shift in focus from nutrigenetics to today's more actionable, behavior change–oriented solutions.

Abrahams highlighted a randomized controlled trial (RCT) carried out in 2015 on the use of glycemic response data to develop personalized nutrition guidance (Zeevi et al., 2015), and a white paper during the same year about the Food4Me study, a web-based RCT on personalized nutrition in seven European countries (Celis-Morales et al., 2017). At the end of that year, she reported, one of the first personalized nutrition companies—which focused on demonstrating effects in terms of behavior change as well as health outcomes—received a large investment, and another company was launched in 2017. By 2018, she said, the personalized nutrition market was gaining steam, and consumer awareness of and interest in its offerings were on the rise.

In 2019, Abrahams launched her own company, Qina, whose aim she described as connecting industry, academia, and health care professionals to ensure an industry focus on science-based solutions with input from practicing providers. She listed a handful of personalized nutrition companies that had been acquired by larger corporations by the end of 2019, and said that in 2020, the COVID-19 pandemic drove consumer interest in and demand for telehealth, smart-eating apps, supplements, and content on how to improve personal health. Another shift occurred at the beginning of 2021, she noted, in terms of the types of solutions offered as well as the business models and partnerships underpinning the offerings.

Abrahams estimated that in 2012, the personalized nutrition market consisted of 16 companies, a number that is now at nearly 400. The industry is highly fragmented, she observed, and difficult to track in terms of both solutions offered and companies' movement within industry segments through partnerships and collaborations (Figure 3-1). Qina was developed, she explained, to help stakeholders navigate and understand the industry by creating a curated database of personalized nutrition solutions. The company helps industry and patient-facing health care professionals understand which solutions are available, what technologies and data points they leverage, who offers them, and which can be integrated.

According to Abrahams, Qina has observed at least four areas in which the number of companies offering a particular type of solution increased between 2014 and 2021: nutritional supplements; microbiome approaches; dietary preference approaches; and devices, including wearables for tracking biologic parameters.

Abrahams next described key aspects of the current personalized nutrition market. She pointed out that the COVID-19 pandemic has increased consumer interest in nutrition-related solutions based in their dietary preferences and health goals, as well as in additional values around which people are personalizing their diets, such as procuring foods locally, choosing organic varieties, and reducing their carbon footprint. She added that companies are increasingly emphasizing behavior change techniques and adding services to their products, such as connections with registered dietitians, to help people implement personalized advice. She noted that the

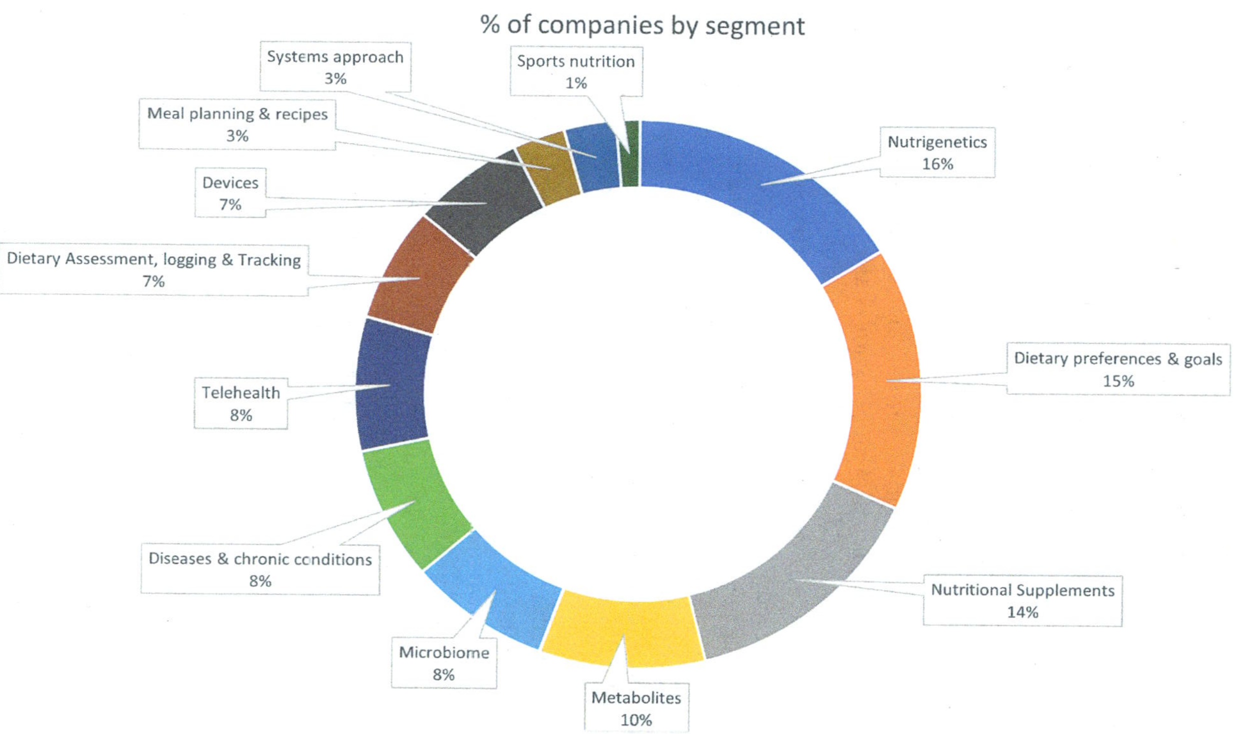

FIGURE 3-1 Breakdown of the personalized nutrition market by segment.
SOURCE: Presented by Mariëtte Abrahams on August 11, 2021.

characteristics of users have also broadened beyond those of the early adopters, explaining that younger consumers are now interested in disease prevention and health optimization, whereas older consumers want to manage and treat symptoms.

As for the corporate structure of the market, Abrahams highlighted an increase in strategic partnerships that she said was driven by the realization that single companies typically are not good at everything, and that teaming could improve the customer experience and provide more value from the data collected. Consumers are demanding more transparency from companies, she observed, including information about the science supporting their products. Companies are no longer focused mainly on funding large clinical trials, she added; they are also interested in data that can inform hyperpersonalization of the delivery and implementation of their services. She cited insights into the optimal interface for consumer interaction and format and frequency for providing information as examples of factors that contribute to consumer success with behavior change.

Abrahams also reviewed key trends in the market, starting with scientific advances driving the development of new solutions. Cardiometabolic health is becoming a driver for new solutions, she observed, and the microbiome is a growing area of focus for many new product launches. She also highlighted the superior outcomes achieved with hybrid approaches that pair personalized nutrition technology with experts who help consumers understand and operationalize the advice they have been given compared with approaches focused mainly on technology. She referenced the earlier perception that the development of sophisticated technology would replace the expertise of health care practitioners. Instead, she argued, it has become clear that such technologies enhance practitioners' effectiveness in supporting patient goals.

Abrahams turned to another trend toward new entrants into the market, such as the pharmaceutical industry. As an example, she cited a German startup's digestive symptom tracking app, which pharmacists recommend to patients who purchase products to treat symptoms of irritable bowel syndrome. Additionally, she pointed to the increasing availability of wider applications of some solutions, such as continuous glucose monitors for patients who do not have diabetes or elevated glucose but are interested in tracking their responses to foods. Lastly, she highlighted a demand for the expertise of health care practitioners both in understanding the science and technologies underlying personalized nutrition and in translating the guidance offered into tailored behavior change strategies for individual patients.

Abrahams next shared her thoughts on the future of personalized nutrition. She identified the concept of food as medicine or food for optimal health as a key focus for future developments. The newest solutions in personalized nutrition are closing the gap between the food and health industries, she observed, with food shopping lists, meal plans, and education being integrated to help patients achieve greater success in following dietary patterns that prevent or treat certain health conditions. Similarly, she described how retailers are playing a larger role in helping consumers improve their health by offering healthy food options and education and in-store guidance to aid them in selecting those foods, wellness services such as biometric screenings, and personalized rewards or discounts. Abrahams cited sustainability as another area of future growth, noting that it is a growing priority for many consumers, fueled by growing interest in food options that are plant-based and produced in environmentally conscience ways. She pointed as well to the emergence of new regulations designed to keep consumers safe as regulators catch up with digital tools. Regulators are giving increasing attention to what types of data are collected by these tools and how they are stored and used, she elaborated, with implications for whether health information being shared on digital platforms is considered medical advice and regulated accordingly.

To conclude her presentation, Abrahams discussed equitable access to personalized nutrition solutions, emphasizing that Qina believes in equity by design. She also suggested that companies should build in levels of product personalization, starting by guiding consumers to credible sources of nutrition education and food literacy or using existing algorithms to provide food-based personalization. Also important, she stressed, is ensuring that the right solutions meet the goals and needs of the relevant population group. She suggested that to this end, companies can use insights into how consumers interact with their products to pair them with solutions they are most likely to use and benefit from. Finally, she highlighted the need for reimbursement for evidence-based solutions for improved health.

Abrahams ended her talk by stating that the personalized nutrition market is dynamic, rapidly growing, and increasingly shifting toward the mainstream, with scientific advances supporting its merits. She added, however, that more could be done to improve inclusivity in research study populations and to provide equitable access to personalized nutrition for a wider consumer base.

THE GENETIC SCALE

Denise Ney, University of Wisconsin–Madison, was the first of three speakers to discuss innovative methodologies and technologies focused on matching nutrition guidance to an individual's genetic makeup. Ney addressed the topic from the angle of population-wide newborn screening for inborn errors of metabolism using whole-exome sequencing (WES). To introduce the topic, she discussed phenylketonuria (PKU), an inborn error of metabolism caused by more than 800 mutations in the gene that produces the enzyme phenylalanine hydroxylase. She described PKU as "the poster child for precision nutrition," given that it exemplifies a condition for which a strong evidence base supports the importance of following a specific diet for a specific genotype. The phenotype of profound cognitive impairment that results from untreated PKU is rare today in the developed world, she observed, because of mandatory newborn screening programs and initiation of a low-phenylalanine diet in affected infants, which was devised in 1953 well before the genetic basis of PKU was understood.

Ney believes newborn screening for inborn errors of metabolism provides an ideal model for evaluating the role of sequencing in population screening. She explained that WES consists of sequencing the protein-coding regions of genes, which are thought to constitute only 1 percent of the genome but to be the location of most known pathogenic mutations. She noted that WES can be compared directly in sensitivity and specificity with tandem mass spectrometry (MS/MS), the established technique for newborn screening programs.

Ney described a recent study on the role of WES in newborn screening for inborn errors of metabolism (Adhikari et al., 2020b), in which the researchers analyzed variants within an exome slice of 78 genes linked with 48 inborn errors of metabolism, ascertained by newborn screening in California using archived dried blood spots from 4.5 million births between 2005 and 2013. Ney emphasized the critical importance of using population-level newborn screening to identify all positive cases of inborn errors of metabolism, many of which are life-threatening, while minimizing false positives to reduce undue stress on families and unnecessary use of medical resources. She explained that MS/MS screening in the study cohort had a sensitivity of 99.0 percent and a specificity of 99.8 percent, which she said is consistent with the quality control standards of the Centers for Disease Control and Prevention for newborn screening programs in the United States. She reported that the sensitivity of WES was 88 percent (571 cases identified, 103 cases missed) overall, but varied among different inborn errors of metabolism. For example, she elaborated, WES detected 100 percent of cases of methylmalonic acidemia caused by known genetic mutations, but only 86 percent of cases of the fatty acid oxidation disorder, very long-chain acyl-CoA dehydrogenase deficiency (VLCADD). According to Ney, the 11 false positives in the study cohort would extrapolate to 8,000 cases per year based on California's birth rate. In contrast, MS/MS yielded 1,362 false positives in 2015. Ney asserted that these results indicate that WES alone is insufficiently sensitive or specific to be the primary screen for most inborn errors of metabolism (Adhikari et al., 2020a).

Ney described another implication of the study: that WES has advantages as a secondary test for infants with abnormal MS/MS screens before further biochemical and clinical studies are undertaken. Elaborating on how WES reduced false positives as a second-tier test, she reported that of 108 false-positive VLCADD cases, WES identified 48 as true negatives, and it identified all 16 of 16 maple syrup urine disease cases as true negatives (Adhikari et al., 2020a). According to Ney, conducting WES in a timely, cost-effective manner could have avoided the cost and family stress of follow-up testing for those inborn errors of metabolism. She added that WES also has the capacity to reveal new genetic variants and to suggest the need for whole-genome sequencing, a diagnostic tool used for critically ill patients with unknown diagnoses.

Jim Kaput, Vydiant, was the second speaker to discuss the genetic scale. He described results from a micronutrient intervention study that assessed genetic contributions to phenotype. Results reported in the first article published by the research team indicated that an individual's genetic ancestry was responsible for at least a portion of baseline levels of vitamin B1 for Europeans, vitamin B12 for Native Americans, and folate for Native Americans (Mathias et al., 2018). Although he characterized these results as important, Kaput said they lack the level of detail needed for application to personalized nutrition guidance.

Because single nucleotide polymorphisms (SNPs) typically do not have effect sizes sufficient for explaining an individual's response to a nutrient or susceptibility to disease, Kaput and his collaborators next pursued assessment of polygenic risk scores (PRSs) (combinations of SNPs) to determine the genetic contribution to vitamin B12 levels. According to Kaput, formal guidelines for assessing multiple variants do not exist, but most groups rely on genome-wide association studies (GWAS)–identified SNPs or SNPs in specific candidate genes. The limitation of this method, he observed, is that GWAS-identified SNPs are based primarily on populations of European descent. To mitigate this limitation, Kaput's research team combined results from genotyping arrays and whole-exome data to identify approximately 7,000 SNPs in 90 genes related to vitamin B12, and then determined the genetic ancestry of each SNP using nearby ancestry informative markers from the Human Genome Diversity Project. They then used an analytical approach to identify 36 SNPs within the genetic pathway of vitamin B12 metabolism that could be used for PRS analysis. PRSs of those SNPs explained 42 percent of phenotypes, Kaput reported, with high PRSs correlating with a preponderance of individuals with high baseline vitamin B12 levels (Fuzo et al., 2021). He added that including other factors known to influence health as covariates (age, sex, body mass index [BMI], Healthy Eating Index score, and mean ancestry components) helped achieve the 42 percent result.

Kaput went on to explain that as a proof of concept for use of PRSs in personalized diets, individuals were stratified into tertiles of PRSs that correlated with plasma vitamin B12 levels. He reported that high PRSs were associated with high baseline vitamin B12 levels, and that individuals in this tercile are therefore at low risk for needing additional vitamin B12, whereas individuals in the middle tercile are at mild risk. Those with the lowest PRSs are at the highest risk for needing additional vitamin B12, a finding that Kaput suggested calls for close monitoring, regular assessment of vitamin B12 levels, and specific dietary recommendations as needed.

In conclusion, Kaput reiterated that assessing multiple genetic variants is more useful than assessing single SNPs for personalizing dietary guidance. It is also important to understand an individual's genetic architecture, he argued, and to adjust associations by incorporating other factors that may influence metabolite levels (e.g., age, sex, dietary intake) as covariates. He suggested that future efforts to replicate his team's results should use the same covariates, adding that some of the SNPs they identified may not appear in other studies that draw on other genetic populations. He asserted that similar analyses will gradually lead to the identification of all SNPs in the vitamin B12 metabolic pathway that are valuable to include and can be considered for use on a genetic population–specific basis.

Ahmed El-Sohemy, University of Toronto and Nutrigenomix Inc., was the third speaker to discuss the genetic scale. He began by observing that genetics and gene products such as enzymes, receptors, and transporters can influence various outcomes related to an individual's response to diet, including sensory perceptions of food, appetite, digestion, absorption, metabolism, and excretion. In El-Sohemy's view, the evidence base is more robust for genetics than for other omics technologies used to provide personalized dietary guidance, but because the availability and strength of evidence vary by genetic marker, it is important to distinguish where recommendations can and cannot be made.

El-Sohemy stated that his research interest is centered on genes that influence responses to nutrients, not disease-associated genes. As an example of the impact of a single SNP on nutrient response, he referenced a 2-year RCT in which a high-protein diet was found to have a stronger effect on reducing body fat and changing body composition among participants versus those without the AA genotype of the fat mass and obesity-associated (FTO) gene (Zhang et al., 2012). The same effect has been replicated in a number of other studies (Antonio et al., 2019; de Luis et al., 2015), he added, including one conducted in a multiethnic population in Toronto (Merritt et al., 2018).

El-Sohemy next reviewed several controversies in the field by addressing six misconceptions that, he said, are often raised by people skeptical of the value of personalizing nutrition guidance based on genetics (Garcia-Bailo and El-Sohemy, 2021). He responded to the first—that single SNPs are useless—by sharing his belief that this criticism comes from genetic association studies that examine specific phenotypes, such as blood levels of vitamin B12 or 25-hydroxy vitamin D. He pointed out, however, that predicting baseline blood levels of a nutrient is different from predicting an individual's response to a dietary intervention based on that nutrient. For example, he said, individuals with low baseline levels of a nutrient might be resistant to increasing dietary intake of that nutrient.

El-Sohemy turned to a second misconception—that people will not change their behaviors—and a third—that more RCT evidence relative to genetics-based dietary guidance is needed. He pointed out that RCT evidence is now available to suggest that giving people certain types of genetic information coupled with actionable recommendations motivates sustainable behavior change (Horne et al., 2020; Nielsen and El-Sohemy, 2014).

El-Sohemy described a fourth misconception—that genetic test results are too complex for people to understand. He agreed that this is likely true if only raw data are provided, but argued that well-designed reports from some testing companies and used by a health care practitioner can help provide practical strategies for needed behavior changes.

El-Sohemy identified as a fifth misconception that family history is more informative than an individual's genetic makeup. He contended that family history alone is only a crude predictor. Families also share common environments, he pointed out, and without an individual's specific genetic information, it is not possible to know which offspring have inherited which combinations of particular genotypes that might affect response to a given dietary intervention.

As a final misconception, El-Sohemy identified the belief that people can simply follow recommendations for healthy eating. He pointed out that some aspects of such guidance could be harmful for some people. To illustrate this point, he explained that approximately 50 percent of the population are "slow" metabolizers of caffeine, and for them following the population-based recommendations for coffee consumption will increase their risk of heart attack, hypertension, and prediabetes.

THE PHYSIOLOGICAL/MICROBIOME SCALE

Sarah Berry, King's College London, was the first of three speakers to discuss innovative methodologies and technologies that focus on matching dietary guidance with an individual at the physiological/microbiome scale. She described the use of big data and novel technologies by PREDICT (Personalized Responses to Dietary Composition Trial) to advance nutrition research and the development of personalized nutrition programs. She explained that PREDICT is an ongoing research collaboration between traditional nutrition academics at King's College London, Massachusetts General Hospital, Stanford University, Harvard Medical School, and Tufts University and a startup technology company, ZOE, that specializes in machine learning and artificial intelligence (AI).

According to Berry, the PREDICT studies aimed to move beyond the constraints of traditional nutrition research in which trade-offs are made between quantity and precision (e.g., high-precision but low-quantity RCTs, or low-precision but large-scale epidemiological studies). She added that PREDICT investigators also seek to capitalize on big data opportunities from new technologies such as digital devices, clinical devices, remote clinical testing, and even citizen science, all of which she said provide data at scale, breadth, depth, and precision. She did not have time to describe in detail all of the studies in the PREDICT program, but highlighted that they all use novel technology and remote home testing and measure the many integrated and interrelated, multidirectional pathways that determine individual responses to dietary intake. She elaborated on the types of methodologies using examples from the PREDICT 1 study.

The PREDICT 1 study's aim, Berry continued, was to use genetic, metabolomic, metagenomic, and meal-context information to predict postprandial responses to food in 1,000 UK participants (main cohort) and 100 U.S. participants (validation cohort). During the baseline clinical visit (study day 1), investigators provided sequential test meals; collected metabolomics, saliva, and urine; conducted genetic testing; took anthropometric measures; monitored blood pressure and heart rate; and administered questionnaires about medical history, lifestyle, and dietary intake. Participants then entered the study's remote, home-based phase (study days 2–14). During this time, Berry reported, participants consumed standardized meals as well as meals of their own choosing; underwent continuous glucose monitoring and monitoring of sleep and physical activity using digital devices; and provided stool samples for microbiome profiling and dried blood spots for measurement of C-peptide, insulin, and triglycerides. They also logged all foods and beverages consumed along with their corresponding satiety levels in an app that was developed by the research team and monitored in real time by a team of nutrition experts who communicated with participants to ensure the provision of complete, high-quality dietary intake data.

Berry illustrated the scale of the PREDICT 1 study data with a series of statistical results, such as 132,000 meals logged, 750,000 metabolomic measures, more than 2 million continuous glucose monitor readings, and 75 billion metagenomic reads. She noted that the amount of data has increased nearly 10-fold now that the PREDICT 2 and 3 studies are complete and recruiting, respectively, and that the PREDICT studies' dataset now includes 40,000 different meal configurations, enabling investigators to consider such factors as the food matrix and nutrient/nutrient interactions. According to Berry, this volume of data enhances study investigators' ability to unravel different exposures related to interindividual variability in outcomes, as indicated by wide variation observed in healthy participants' responses in triglyceride and glucose levels after consumption of a standardized meal in a tightly controlled setting, for example (Berry et al., 2020). She listed exposures of interest, including meal composition, meal context (time of day, meal sequence), genetics, microbiome, age and sex, blood pressure, and habitual diet, as well as outcomes of interest, including metabolomics, microbiome composition, glycemic control, inflammation, endothelial dysfunction, and hunger and energy intake. She cited serum measures and anthropometry as two examples of factors that are both exposures and outcomes.

Berry next shared a broad overview of PREDICT 1's results, emphasizing that meal composition and context are as important as such factors as age and genetics in determining an individual's response to food intake. For each outcome, the investigators explored the relative contribution of different exposures and found that the importance of a given exposure was different depending on the outcome (Figure 3-2). Berry explained that PREDICT 1 also identified microbiome signatures (i.e., compositions of microbes) that were associated either with healthy dietary habits and favorable health markers or with unhealthy diets and unfavorable health markers.

Berry then described how ZOE used the PREDICT 1 results to create a machine learning model that uses an individual's results from an at-home test to predict his or her responses to food, and then delivers personalized dietary guidance. The at-home test includes a microbiome assessment, which allows for additional personalized guidance to consume either a gut booster or suppressor. As for the future of the ZOE PREDICT program, Berry stated that the research team is "sitting on a goldmine of data" and has only just scratched the surface of its potential to yield new insights and lead to additional, more stratified, and personalized nutrition solutions.

Michal Rein, Weizmann Institute of Science and University of Haifa (Israel), was the second speaker to discuss the physiologic/microbiome scale. She described an approach to personalized nutrition guidance involving prediction of glycemic responses using clinical and microbiome features. Recounting a study conducted 9 years earlier, Rein explained that researchers continuously tracked glucose levels and multiple other clinical, lifestyle, diet, and microbiome measures among 1,000 healthy individuals. They measured 2-hour postprandial glucose responses (PPGRs) (changes in blood glucose levels during the 2 hours following a meal), a metric that Rein said is associated with risk for such outcomes as metabolic diseases, diabetes, and weight gain.

The study produced data on approximately 2 million PPGRs for 50,000 meals consumed by participants, Rein reported, and revealed high interindividual variation in PPGR to the same meal. Responses were reproducible within participants, she elaborated, indicating that they are highly personalized and can be predicted accurately. She described how the researchers used these results along with participants' clinical and microbiome data to

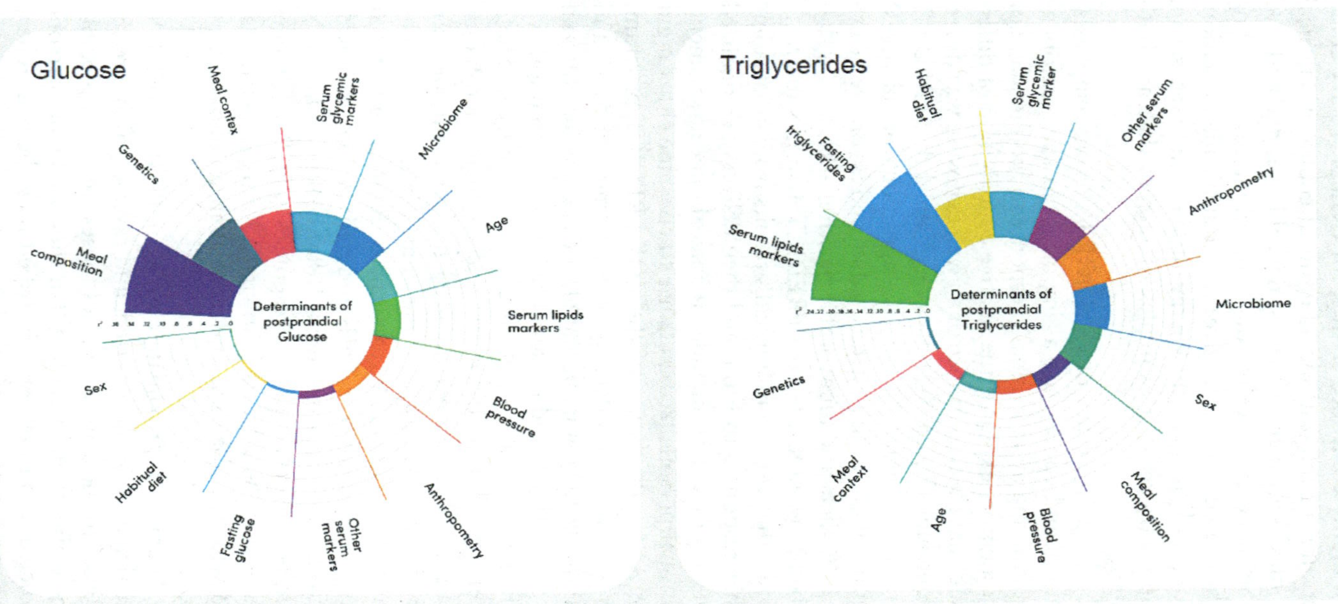

FIGURE 3-2 Differences in the relative contributions of exposures to the outcomes of blood levels of glucose (left) and triglycerides (right) in PREDICT 1 study participants.
SOURCE: Presented by Sarah Berry on August 11, 2021.

develop a machine learning algorithm that accurately predicted personalized PPGRs to any food combination. A short-term intervention tested the effects of personalized dietary intervention based on the algorithm, she added, and indicated that the personalized diets lowered PPGR in people with prediabetes (Zeevi et al., 2015).

Rein discussed the next phase of this work, which was to assess the clinical impact of a personalized postprandial targeting (PPT) diet. She shared three interventions that tested a PPT diet, beginning with a study conducted in participants with impaired glucose tolerance (i.e., prediabetes). The 225 participants were randomly assigned to a PPT diet or a Mediterranean diet, the commonly recommended diet for prediabetes, and instructed to follow the diet (without restrictions on calories consumed) for 6 months and to undergo additional follow-up for another 6 months. Continuous glucose monitoring and recording of dietary intake continued throughout the 6-month intervention. Rein reported that the PPT diet decreased daily time with high glucose levels and reduced hemoglobin A1c levels compared with the Mediterranean diet, and the researchers concluded that the PPT diet improves glycemic control and metabolic parameters in individuals with prediabetes (Ben-Yacov et al., 2021).

Next, Rein continued, the researchers conducted a pilot study in which 16 participants with newly diagnosed type 2 diabetes who were not taking any glucose-lowering medications were instructed to follow a PPT diet for 6 months. They observed changes in gut microbiome composition associated with improved fasting blood glucose levels, as well as a reduction in hemoglobin A1c levels. Finally, Rein showed that the PPT diet induced diabetes remission in more than 60 percent of participants.

Rein then presented a third, ongoing intervention performed by the company DayTwo, which is testing an algorithm-based dietary intervention in a multicenter dietary modification project among 251 participants with type 2 diabetes taking glucose-lowering medications. She reported that following the diet decreased hemoglobin A1c in more than 80 percent of the participants, and also reduced body weight an average of 4 percent. Thirty percent of participants also self-reported reduced use of glucose-lowering medication after 3–4 months of intervention.

The results of these three interventions, Rein said in summary, support the use of personalized dietary interventions for improving glycemic control and metabolic health.

Guru Banavar, Viome, was the panel's third speaker. Building on the prior speakers' discussion of genetics as the basis for understanding glycemic response and other metabolic effects on biology, he stated that gene expression (i.e., the RNA molecules that are produced and transcribed by one's genome and ultimately control the development of chronic disease) can also be modulated with diet and lifestyle. To illustrate this concept, he explained that *C. diff* colitis, an inflammation of the colon caused by *Clostridioides* bacteria, does not necessarily develop simply when those bacteria are present; rather, the infection begins when the host organism starts to express certain genes that result in illness.

Banavar cited two key technologies that Viome uses to create personalized food and supplement recommendations based on the premise of dietary modulation of gene expression. He described the first, metatranscriptomics, as measurement and detection of RNA molecules across a range of organisms, from microbes to humans. Viome has a scalable platform for extracting RNA data from a user's stool sample, he said, which are then fed into the second key technology, AI and machine learning, to generate personalized recommendations.

Banavar contended that, based on Viome's research, genetic expression as measured by RNA molecules is superior to genetics for making dietary recommendations. He has used these data to predict differences in individuals' glycemic response to foods such that single foods can be classified as "enjoy" or "minimize" for a given individual. Furthermore, he continued, Viome has layered gut microbiome pathway analysis onto the glycemic response data to further classify specific foods as "super," "enjoy," "minimize," or "avoid" for a given individual. Banavar explained that the gut microbiome is responsible for producing metabolites (e.g., butyrate) that influence an individual's response to foods and for eliminating compounds (e.g., oxalate) that are not beneficial.

Banavar then illustrated Viome's use of glycemic response data plus microbiome pathway analysis to develop personalized dietary guidance, taking spinach as an example. Although spinach likely evokes a low glycemic response and is typically recommended as a healthy food for everyone, he observed, it is also high in oxalates. He explained that for individuals with high microbiome pathway activity for oxalate elimination, spinach could be a "super" food, but that it could be less beneficial and even raise risk for negative health outcomes (e.g., kidney stones) among individuals with low microbiome pathway activity for oxalate elimination.

Banavar next highlighted Viome's efforts to feed phenotypic and gene expression data from its hundreds of thousands of customers into its AI engine not only to generate insights for personalized nutrition recommendations but also to detect certain key initial signals of chronic disease. The company has launched a discovery program around this concept, he explained, and is considering a variety of therapeutic areas, including metabolic, gastrointestinal, and oncologic. As an example of the power of RNA-based discovery using large-scale data, Banavar noted that Viome recently received a U.S. Food and Drug Administration (FDA) breakthrough device designation for a biomarker that is useful for diagnosing early-stage oral and throat cancer.

Looking forward, Banavar envisioned the potential to use RNA detection combined with AI analysis to examine host/microbiome interactions. This systems biology approach has the potential to detect specific molecular signatures associated with defined pathogenic processes, he explained, which can lead to predictive, diagnostic, prognostic, and therapeutic clinical applications.

THE INDIVIDUAL SCALE

Andres Acosta, Mayo Clinic, was the first of three speakers to discuss innovative methodologies and technologies for developing personalized nutrition approaches tailored to an individual in terms of both physiology and behavior. He discussed the use of pathophysiological and behavioral phenotypes for guiding obesity management to enhance weight loss.

Forty percent of U.S. adults have obesity, Acosta said, and obesity is a risk factor for numerous chronic diseases, as well as premature death. He reported that, despite U.S. spending of $480 billion in direct annual health care costs on obesity (Waters and Graf, 2018) and the availability of five FDA-approved medications, five devices, three bariatric surgery options, and countless lifestyle programs for weight management, the prevalence of adult obesity continues to rise. Furthermore, he contended, these "one-size-fits-all" obesity treatment approaches are not working, and he proposed that a "precision obesity" approach (to include a precision nutrition component) is essential.

Acosta then elaborated on the shortcomings of existing obesity treatment approaches, pointing to the considerable heterogeneity among patients in how much weight they lose in response to a given treatment, whether lifestyle-, drug-, device-, or surgery-based (Figure 3-3).

Similar heterogeneity exists among patients in traits related to energy balance, he reported, highlighting as an example the wide variation in the number of calories consumed by individual patients before they reached maximal fullness. He added that patients show similar variability in post-prandial fullness (i.e., how full a patient feels 2 hours after a meal) and resting energy expenditure (Acosta et al., 2015). Current obesity classifications are based on a patient's risk of obesity-associated comorbidities (Lewis et al., 2009; Lonardo et al., 2020), Acosta pointed out, instead of stratifying patients with obesity based on prediction of their response to various treatments.

The way obesity is traditionally viewed, Acosta continued, is that phenotypes drive the disease, for which drugs are then developed, and outcomes are highly variable among patients. In contrast, he said, a precision medicine approach starts with the disease and then segments it into various phenotypes with their own unique developmental pathways, an approach

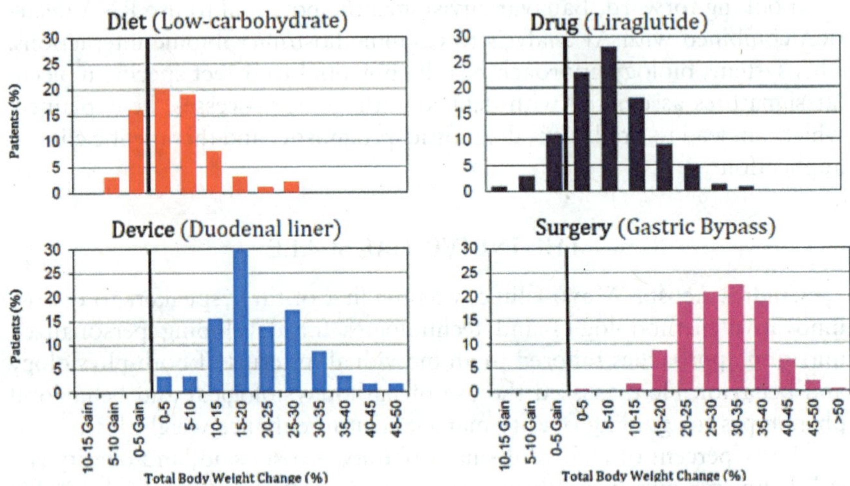

FIGURE 3-3 Weight loss in response to different obesity treatment interventions varies widely among patients.
SOURCES: Presented by Andres Acosta on August 11, 2021; Kaplan, 2017. Reprinted with permission from Lee M. Kaplan.

that leads to targeted treatments that result in better patient outcomes. He noted that an individual's phenotype is determined by the interaction of genomics, which indicates diseases to which the person may be predisposed, with such environmental and lifestyle factors as diet, physical activity, and other exposures.

Acosta next explained that obesity phenotypes have been proposed on the basis of their pathophysiology. For context, he explained that obesity results from an imbalance between an individual's energy intake and energy expenditure. Intake is driven mainly by hunger, satiation, satiety, and emotional eating, he elaborated, whereas expenditure is driven by resting energy expenditure, exercise, and nonexercise activity thermogenesis. The Mayo Clinic phenotypes patients with obesity based on their results on a series of tests measuring domains that influence energy intake and expenditure. Specifically, Acosta explained, patients arrive for testing after an overnight fast and undergo measurement of body composition and resting energy expenditure. Next, they consume a standardized meal with a radiolabeled isotope that enables assessment of their gastric emptying, and they are also assessed in terms of appetite, hunger, satiation, satisfaction, and emotional eating. Four hours later, patients are presented with an *ad libitum* meal and instructed to consume as much as they wish. The number of calories they consume before feeling full is measured, and they are followed for another

2 hours to assess satisfaction and fullness. In addition, Acosta said, patients record the number of steps they take and their exercise levels (Acosta et al., 2021).

After conducting this series of tests with more than 500 patients, Acosta explained, the Mayo Clinic applied machine learning to the resulting data to identify four obesity phenotypes (Acosta et al., 2015). The first, hungry brain, occurs when a patient consumes excessive amounts of calories on a given eating occasion. The problem is abnormal satiation, which Acosta described as a problem in the brain. The second phenotype is hungry gut, where the problem is abnormal postprandial satiety. Acosta noted that these patients feel full after consuming a reasonable number of calories, but feel hungry again relatively soon thereafter. The third type is emotional hunger, in which people eat in response to positive and/or negative emotions, and the fourth type is slow burn, characterized by an abnormal metabolism. When distribution of the four obesity phenotypes was measured in 450 new patients (Figure 3-4), Acosta reported, around one-quarter of patients had more than one phenotype, and about 15 percent had none of the four.

Acosta stated that, since identifying the four main obesity phenotypes in 2015, the Mayo Clinic has completed multiple proof-of-concept, placebo-controlled trials to demonstrate that phenotypes can help enhance weight loss in patients with obesity. The trials have evaluated response to

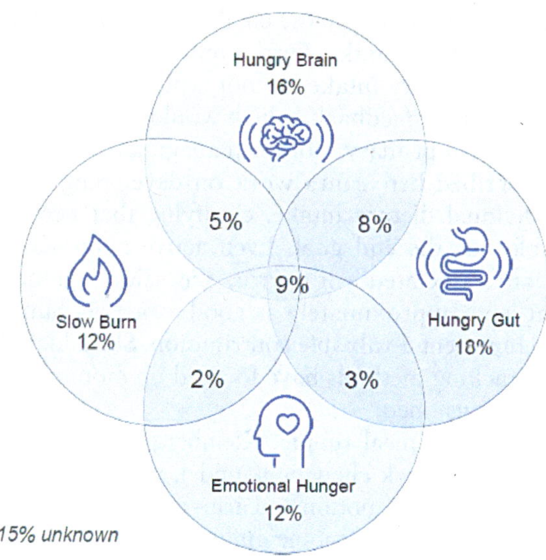

FIGURE 3-4 Distribution of obesity phenotypes in 450 patients.
SOURCES: Presented by Andres Acosta on August 11, 2021; modified from Acosta, et al., 2021. Reprinted with permission from John Wiley and Sons.

obesity pharmacotherapy and endoscopic devices, he explained, adding that phenotype-guided pharmacotherapy in clinical practice can almost double the amount of weight loss at 12 months from baseline compared with standard use of pharmacotherapy (Acosta et al., 2021).

Going forward, Acosta said, the researchers will continue to examine the deeper phenotypes underlying an individual's primary obesity phenotype, using multiomics in an effort to predict phenotypes and identify their underlying causes. He predicted that additional research will also enhance understanding of whether the four phenotypes are causes or consequences of obesity, and indicate whether additional obesity phenotypes may exist or even whether fewer than four phenotypes are necessary for finding the right intervention for the right patient. He predicted further that in the future, it will be possible to measure phenotypes with a simple blood test, and that this will become a routine companion diagnosis helping to improve treatment outcomes for people with obesity.

Samantha Kleinberg, Stevens Institute of Technology, discussed technology-based monitoring of individual dietary intake. She began by stating that current approaches to tracking dietary intake require active input, in contrast to passive approaches that are common for measuring such biometrics as sleep and physical activity. Even with digital approaches to tracking dietary intake, she pointed out, individuals still must remember to take photos and/or complete questionnaires about meals consumed, for example, and are often limited by the challenges associated with complete and accurate recall of food intake. Furthermore, she observed, existing approaches to tracking dietary intake are not typically structured to provide individuals with real-time feedback, which would be particularly useful for those who use diet as a primary tool for managing disease.

Kleinberg described her team's work on developing passive methods for tracking individual dietary intake, clarifying that perfect accuracy is neither attainable nor the end goal. Even active approaches to tracking dietary intake are associated with error, she said, arguing that passive approaches that were approximately as good as active, human-driven approaches would represent a valuable contribution. She added that efforts to develop passive tracking methods have focused on monitoring when meals occur and what is consumed.

In terms of tracking meal timing, Kleinberg reported that audio sensors (e.g., earbuds that track chewing sounds), motion sensors (e.g., other wearables that measure head motion and arm- and wrist-to-mouth motions), and multimodal sensors that combine audio and motion have been tested. She explained that multimodal sensors can help overcome the limitations of sensors that pick up only sounds or motions, but she acknowledged that even multimodal tools for tracking meal timing provide insufficient information for tracking specific intake, let alone developing personalized guidance.

With respect to efforts to track the specific foods people eat, Kleinberg pointed out that until recently most of this work has occurred in laboratory settings using individual sensors to measure audio or motion or to record images of meals consumed. Multimodal sensors provide more complete data relative to single-mode sensors for tracking foods consumed, she affirmed, but said that her lab's data suggest that combining multiple types of single-mode sensors is not necessary; rather, one type of motion plus one type of audio sensor is sufficient. In lab settings, she continued, each chew and swallow is recorded and labeled, whereas this level of assessment is not possible in free-living environments. But by combining data from lab and free-living environments, she suggested, it may be possible to identify types of foods consumed in an automated way. She reported that in the lab setting, researchers in one study correctly identified each bite of food by type (e.g., steak, potato, or salad) with 83 percent accuracy (Mirtchouk et al., 2019). A similar degree of accuracy was measured in free-living environments, she noted, and incorporating these data also improved the accuracy (to 88 percent) of lab-collected data (Mirtchouk et al., 2019).

Kleinberg observed that major gaps remain despite advances in passive methods for tracking meal timing and type. She explained that these methods do not provide information about why, when, and what people eat; their levels of hunger and fullness; or the social and emotional context in which eating occurs. She also identified this as another major limitation on the generalizability of the information obtained, because although passive methods can reliably classify intake for 40 or 50 different types of foods (e.g., salad, soup, cookies), the same types of food may vary considerably in composition across cultures and countries.

Looking ahead, Kleinberg predicted that more reasonably priced wearables for audio and motion tracking of food intake will become available in the next 5 years. She added that the level of specificity needed for categorizing foods using these tools depends on the intended use of the data. For example, she said, if the goal is to understand food sensitivities without using an elimination diet, specific foods need to be identified, something that could be achieved by combining self-reported dietary intake with data from wearables. On the other hand, if the goal is to track macronutrient intake, less specificity and contrast will be required, and only one type of sensor (audio or motion) may need to be worn.

Diana Thomas, United States Military Academy at West Point, was the panel's third speaker. Thomas emphasized the richness of data collected via open-ended, free-form survey questions and analyzed with natural language processing software. She noted that nutrition surveys typically ask multiple-choice or Likert-style questions whereby participants select from a continuum of responses, for reasons related mainly to perceived ease of analysis. According to Thomas, it is not necessarily easier to analyze the latter responses, and current statistical software is equipped to assess and extract a wealth of information from free-form text survey response data.

Thomas illustrated the value of such data with an example from a survey on weight bias. Of 26 survey questions, only one requested a free-form text response: "In your opinion, what does the American public think about people with obesity?" Assessment of sentiment is one of the first approaches statisticians take to analyze free-form text, Thomas explained, with support from statistical software packages that have built-in dictionaries that assign various levels of positive or negative sentiment levels to different words and classify words according to emotions (Thomas et al., 2020). In this example survey, mostly negative sentiments were detected in response to the above question, Thomas reported, and more people responded with words that fell into the category of disgust relative to any other emotion (Figure 3-5).

When the sentiment data were combined with the survey's Likert-style question asking respondents to classify their self-perceived weight status, sentiment became more negative as the respondent's self-perceived weight status grew heavier, Thomas reported. She reiterated that this combination of data from Likert-style, multiple-choice questions and free-form text data provided a depth of insight beyond that gained from either type of question alone.

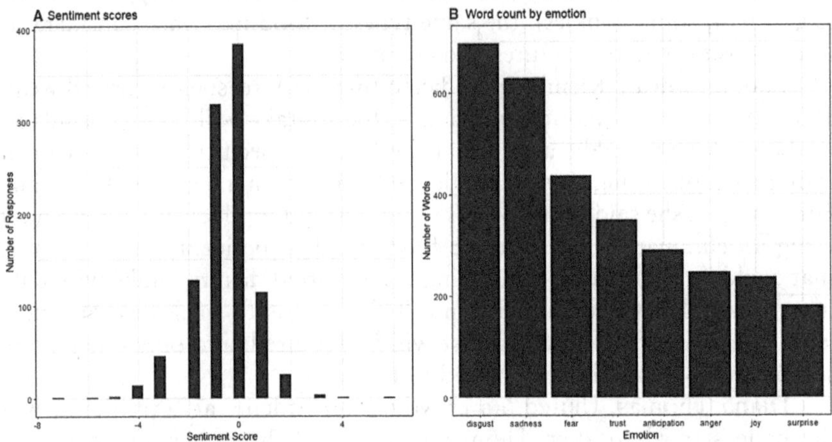

FIGURE 3-5 Measures of sentiment and emotion in response to a survey question about the American public's perception of people with obesity.
SOURCES: Presented by Diana Thomas on August 11, 2021; Thomas et al., 2020. Reprinted with permission from John Wiley and Sons.

THE SOCIAL-ECOLOGIC SCALE

Kayla de la Haye, University of Southern California, discussed innovations in research on the social and ecological settings in which people access and consume food. Eating behaviors are particularly susceptible to social and environmental influences, de la Haye began, because they are habitual and often shaped unconsciously by proximal cues. She pointed out, for example, that eating companions encode social rules and social resources that can enable or constrain the food choices of those eating with them (Delormier et al., 2009). She maintained that achieving dietary behavior change depends on both personal agency and supportive social and environmental structures. When people exert personal choice and effort to change eating behaviors, she asserted, those new healthful habits will be difficult to sustain if they are embedded in unsupportive structures. She stressed further that people with low incomes and those in communities of color are unequally exposed to structural influences that do not support healthy eating.

de la Haye discussed the use of new sources of social data and network science to understand more precisely how social exposures and social networks influence what people eat. Findings indicate that people are eating in increasingly diverse settings with diverse eating partners, she reported, as they eat food away from home more often, have fewer family meals, and eat with a greater variety of people in their social networks (Koehly and Loscalzo, 2009). Reflecting on her ongoing research, she stated that people tend to eat with about one-quarter of the approximately 20 people closest to them in their social network, although those eating networks vary across people and populations. Longitudinal social network research using network analytic methods has shown that nutritional health and people's social networks are interdependent, she continued, because people tend to select and form social ties with people who are similar to themselves (Centola, 2011; de la Haye et al., 2011; McPherson et al., 2001; Valente et al., 2009). She added that research has linked these patterns to several contributing factors, including homophily, propinquity, and stigma: homophily is a phenomenon whereby people connect with others who have similar characteristics, such as ethnicity, socioeconomic status, or health risks and inequalities; propinquity is the tendency to connect with others who are geographically close; and stigma drives the exclusion of individuals and groups based on stigmatized traits.

In addition to these social selection processes, de la Haye cited strong evidence that social networks influence people's health behaviors, including eating behaviors, through such mechanisms of social influence as mimicry and normative influence, as well as by providing social support (Aral and Nicolaides, 2017; Fletcher et al., 2011; Trogdon et al., 2008; Valente et al., 2009; Zhang et al., 2018). She gave the example of a study in which adolescents with friends who frequently ate energy-dense, low-nutrient junk foods were found to be likely to increase their intake of these foods over the course of one school year. She added that this effect of social network influence was significant after controlling for whom the teens selected as friends, their own beliefs about junk foods, and their demographics (de la Haye et al., 2013).

Overall, de la Haye summarized, these dynamics of social selection, social influence, and corresponding shared exposures influence diet and health such that people with the greatest nutritional health risks are more likely to find themselves in social networks that also confer health risks. She emphasized that these social exposures reinforce and influence nutritional health behaviors, and can be barriers to behavior change or targeted in network interventions.

de la Haye next described two types of intervention approaches that use social networks to promote health behavior change. The first is segmentation, which targets at-risk social groups (e.g., family or peer groups) rather than individuals as promoters of positive social influence, norms, and support for healthy habits (Valente, 2012). A second strategy is alteration, in which an intervention is crafted to change people's social networks by building new, adjacent health network ties (e.g., through intentional group or buddy activities) that can increase access to positive social influences, norms, and support (Valente, 2012).

Lastly, de la Haye described as another opportunity to improve eating habits the use of new methods and data to better understand the food environments to which people are exposed. Her group is currently using big data from mobility traces (smartphone-captured information about geolocation) to analyze the daily movements of large populations over time, including patterns of exposure to specific food environments and visits to food outlets. In the future, de la Hayes predicted, this type of data will be able to inform tailored interventions that, for example, might intervene in real time to help people make healthy choices in certain food environments to which they are exposed.

Concluding, de la Haye summarized two opportunities to pursue personal and precision nutrition for all populations. She described first the use of innovations in data, data science, and behavioral and social science to gain both more precise insights into the social and built environments where people acquire and eat food and richer knowledge of how social-ecological mechanisms influence diets. As the second opportunity, she identified the application of these findings to develop precision nutrition knowledge and interventions that will be effective, actionable, and equitable.

Sean Duffy, Omada Health, shared examples of his company's insights illustrating how virtual care can be used to improve health behaviors. As a first example, he explained that when members join Omada, they are asked what challenges they expect to face as they try to change their health behaviors, such as eating and physical activity. The answers they give, he said, provide helpful context as members begin to develop a relationship with their Omada coach and care team. He added that the verb tenses used in the responses provide additional insight. Responses in the present tense—for example, "I hate to cook" or "I don't enjoy many vegetables"—are correlated with less weight loss, whereas responses in the past tense—for example, "I used to eat extra portions of sweets"—are correlated with more weight loss. Omada characterized the latter responses as framing a "growth mindset" in which intelligence and talent are viewed as more flexible and changeable.

A second insight, Duffy continued, is that the combination of technology and human support appears to enhance accountability and influence subtle changes in behavior. As an example, he described how when coaches engaged directly with members after noticing that they exhibited unconscious behavioral patterns, the behavior of meal tracking increased to almost the same level as that obtained through automatic nudges, and more weight loss was achieved. Duffy attributed the improvement to the human touchpoint and outreach of care and support.

Based on that insight, Duffy said, Omada developed a strategy for sending members personalized nudges that it calls "coach plays," in which the program's coaches identify patterns of member behavior and respond with suggestions for improvements. He described two food-related examples. In one, a coach notices a member tracking the same breakfast several days in a row and suggests ideas for small substitutions that maintain similar flavors but increase the nutritional quality of the meal. In the other, the coach notices that a member has not mentioned a particular type of food in the past month of meal logs and suggests how the member might enjoy that food in future meals. Omada has observed modifications in user behaviors and improved member–coach rapport, Duffy reported, within 2 weeks of these types of coach plays.

Michael Howell, Google, reviewed three categories of publicly available, anonymized, and aggregated datasets that are useful for public health research. The first is aggregated, anonymized search queries, which, he explained can provide insights into people's information needs and how those needs change over time. As an example, he showed how the Google Trends tool illustrated a sharp increase in interest in COVID-19 between January and March 2020. As the pandemic evolved, Google made available two additional search query datasets: COVID-19 Search Symptoms (geographic trends in searches for specific health symptoms) and COVID-19 Vaccine Search Insights (trends from searches for topics related to COVID-19 vaccines, such as safety and side effects).

As a second category of Google datasets to support public health efforts, Howell described maps that can aid in understanding distance and how it relates to travel time, which he explained can provide information about built environments. As an example, he shared a research article comparing global differences in travel time to health care facilities by car and by walking, which included a color-coded map to quickly convey differences among regions (Weiss et al., 2020). Another example of the use of distance and travel time data is the COVID-19 Vaccination Access dataset, which Howell noted has been used by Boston Children's Hospital and Ariadne Labs to identify "vaccine deserts" and to calculate travel time to vaccine locations from various starting points.[1]

The third category of anonymized, aggregated datasets described by Howell is community mobility. An example of this dataset's application is research examining how many people traveled from one zip code to another during a given period of time, which he said was used to develop a hierarchical organization of urban mobility and its connection with city livability (Bassolas et al., 2019). He noted that community mobility data have also been used to assess trends in movement to various destinations during the COVID-19 pandemic. He illustrated this function with a real-time example showing that at the time of the workshop, Santa Clara County (California) was 51 percent below baseline for movement to workplaces but only 10 percent below baseline for movement to grocery and pharmacy locations.

PANEL DISCUSSION

Promoting Health Equity

Responding to a question about how the personalized nutrition industry can avoid targeting a narrow segment of consumers at the cost of equity, Abrahams asserted that companies with values centered on improving the health of all consumers tend to partner with like-minded companies. They also seek inputs from health care professionals, she added, about incorporating equity at the front end of product and service designs.

Replying to a question about how to ensure the collection of adequately diverse data for the development of personalized advice across a broad spectrum of the population, Berry offered two comments. First, she proposed the use of novel approaches to recruiting people for such research, aimed at making participation as accessible as possible for diverse populations. Second, she argued that personalized nutrition is at a transition point at which it is creating large-scale, high-depth data and can apply those data in a stratified way that can be more broadly accessible. With continued

---

[1] See Vaccine Equity Planner, available at https://vaccineplanner.org (accessed October 11, 2021).

learning, she predicted, it will be possible to identify key dietary factors that are important for an individual based on a few simple attributes.

Banavar noted that Viome has made a breakthrough in reducing the cost of RNA sequencing to less than $100, which he estimated to be affordable for most U.S. consumers. He predicted that in the next few years, further advances could make this technology affordable for middle-class populations in developing countries, and that eventually the costs could decrease even more. He proposed shifting the focus from the cost of the technology to its value in terms of health advantages it can provide.

Reimbursement for Personalized Nutrition Solutions

According to Kaput, it is necessary to apply machine learning to integrate more data across multiple scales (e.g., genetic, microbiome) in order to grow the evidence base to a point that it can support reimbursement for more personalized nutrition solutions. Payers will want to see a return on their investment, El-Sohemy added, and he suggested that it would be helpful to have economic analyses demonstrating that investments in personalized nutrition solutions can be cost-saving in the longer term.

Duffy explained that Omada members do not self-pay; the company approaches payers to request that they cover the Omada solution based on its demonstrated value in clinical and economic studies. He noted that for nearly 10 percent of commercially insured U.S. adults, at least some part of Omada membership is a fully covered benefit, coded as a preventive benefit and bypassing deductible and coinsurance payments. Omada has focused on the commercial insurance market to date, he added, but in the future wants its services to be covered by all types of health insurance policies.

Addressing Potential Biases in Computational Methods Used to Develop Personalized Solutions

Howell commented that although technologies such as machine learning are powerful, they have limitations, such as the inability to fully address the different types of bias associated with their multiscale data inputs. In Banavar's view, a key approach to addressing bias is increasing a study's sample size and ensuring that its design incorporates participants with diverse phenotypes. He suggested that sample sizes exceeding 100,000 and capturing phenotypes from 70 or 80 countries are representative across the human population and fundamentally help to reduce bias. Berry and Rein agreed, and Berry added that a challenge is recruiting participants from a broader demographic than the "worried well" population that tends to volunteer for nutrition research studies and/or purchase personalized nutrition products.

Banavar also maintained that collecting real-world evidence is critical for improving the usefulness of computational methods. Initial training of an AI or machine learning system is constrained by the training dataset he observed, but it is important that continuous learning and updates to the model occur as the dataset grows with the addition of real-world evidence. Berry added that as datasets grow, researchers would do well to evolve their processes and algorithms accordingly, and to announce that their advice has also evolved based on the availability of additional information.

Acosta urged testing of processes in unsupervised as well as supervised settings (i.e., clinical trials), so that both critical reasoning and empirical validation can be applied. Thomas pointed out that a limitation of natural language processing is that sentiment dictionaries are human-made and do not necessarily capture all nuances of current trends in the use of certain words and phrases; therefore, researchers must review the data manually and ask whether the results of applying natural language processing make sense in the overall context of a participant's responses. Machine learning cannot indicate definitively what is going on, she stressed, reiterating the importance of applying a human element to data analysis.

Using Technology to Provide Insight into Social-Ecological Contexts

de la Haye observed that the suite of data sources now available, such as those in Google, provides the opportunity to gain understanding of populations and their exposures across various levels of social factors and built environments. The ability to analyze these kinds of data at the large-population scale is particularly exciting, she argued, as it allows for identification of differences in exposures and disease risk across populations. Such insights may become apparent only after repeated exposures over months or even years, she noted, giving these data sources advantages over smaller, shorter-term studies that would be less likely to pick up those signals.

Involving Social Networks and Communities in Research Designs

de la Haye observed that community-based participatory research approaches are increasingly being used for social network and ecological-focused interventions. These approaches, she elaborated, draw on local community organizations and families as key networks of people who are open to helping with intervention planning and creating social and community-level change. She stated that the availability of stakeholder and participant networks is critical in setting the stage for policy and environmental change interventions to be successful and sustainable.

Duffy described his vision for Omada's ability to help answer the research community's questions regarding personalized nutrition, which includes enrolling a large-enough membership base to serve as the source for recruiting participants for large-scale RCTs. He also stressed that personalized nutrition guidance must be aligned with an individual's ability and willingness to change behavior, and suggested that technology could provide "digital trails" to facilitate behavior change.

4

Implementation of Precision and Personalized Nutrition

Presenters in this session of the workshop provided academic, regulatory, and industry perspectives on opportunities and challenges in the implementation of precision and personalized nutrition. Robin McKinnon, U.S. Food and Drug Administration (FDA), moderated the session's six presentations and an ensuing panel discussion.

WILL PRECISION NUTRITION HELP IN ACHIEVING GREATER HEALTH EQUITY?

Christina Roberto, University of Pennsylvania, discussed challenges to the potential of precision nutrition to achieve greater health equity. She began by disclosing that her answer to the question in her presentation's title was a skeptical "maybe." Roberto stressed that precision nutrition has tremendous potential to offer people targeted guidance based on their individual disease risks and biological responses to diet. At the same time, she asserted, while the idea of being able to provide tailored nutrition advice to individuals is appealing, doing so requires understanding the complex interplay among biological factors, food environments, and other systems-level forces that affect health (Rodgers and Collins, 2020). Although these factors are acknowledged in discussions of precision nutrition, she argued, those conversations tend to focus on individual-level factors. Roberto emphasized the importance of broader thinking because those factors interact with many environmental- and systems-level forces that influence food choices.

Roberto provided an example of environmental- and systems-level effects via maps indicating differences in life expectancy in different neighborhoods of Philadelphia. She pointed to 20-year gaps in life expectancy between some neighborhoods distinguished by income levels and population demographics.[1] These gaps are not all diet-driven, she maintained, but diet-related chronic diseases contribute to disproportionate rates of chronic disease and mortality in low-income neighborhoods. According to Roberto, this observation highlights the importance of applying precision nutrition in a way that does not widen income and racial/ethnic disparities.

Roberto described "a vicious cycle of unhealthy dietary habits" whereby environmental drivers of food intake exploit biological, psychosocial, and social and economic vulnerabilities that contribute to overconsumption of unhealthy foods, driving preferences and demand for those foods (Roberto et al., 2015). She pointed out that nearly two-thirds of U.S. adults have a diet-related chronic disease, and many people do not adhere to dietary recommendations—even simple messages, such as "eat more fruits and vegetables"—that have been consistent for decades. On a scale of 0–100, where 100 indicates adherence to all food group and nutrient intake components of the *Dietary Guidelines for Americans*, Americans have fluctuated between a score of 56 and 60 each year since at least 2005 (USDA and HHS, 2020). Roberto expressed her doubt that targeted nutrition advice will solve that problem because lack of knowledge is not the only and often not the main barrier to healthful eating.

Roberto discussed the challenges of communicating nutrition messages to the public and achieving behavior change. Beginning with an explanation from basic psychology, she highlighted that people have limited memories and that it takes effort to process information. She explained that psychologists tend to think about two systems with which people think and make decisions and judgments: system 1 comprises fast, automatic, effortless actions based on associations and emotions; system 2 comprises slow, controlled, effortful actions based on reason and logic (Kahneman, 2003). She pointed out that most food decisions are made with system 1 and shared a research example to illustrate human limitations in terms of recalling and implementing nutrition messages.

In Roberto's example, researchers assessed the memorability and actionability of the personalized guideline from the 2005 food pyramid ("MyPyramid"), which a person could generate from a website to learn

---

[1] From *Mapping Life Expectancy: Philadelphia*, available here: https://societyhealth.vcu.edu/work/the-projects/mapsphiladelphia.html (accessed October 11, 2021).

how many servings from each food group should be eaten daily (Ratner and Riis, 2014). They compared MyPyramid with the Half Plate Guideline, a simple message instructing people to fill half their plate with fruits and vegetables. Study subjects were first assessed for their motivation to follow nutritional guidelines, and were then randomized to view either the MyPyramid or Half Plate message. When asked to provide open-ended recall immediately after viewing the message, Roberto reported, 85 and 19 percent, respectively, recalled Half Plate and MyPyramid perfectly. Motivation to follow the Half Plate Guideline was higher than motivation to follow MyPyramid among both the low- and high-motivated groups as assessed at baseline. When the study was replicated and outcomes were assessed 1 month later, Roberto continued, 62 and 0.7 percent, respectively, recalled the recommended food group servings in Half Plate and MyPyramid correctly (Riis and Ratner, 2011). In Roberto's view, a key takeaway from this research is that simple guidelines have tremendous recall advantages. She acknowledged that the recall burden is reduced with technologies that can remind people of advice they have been given, but expressed concern about increasing population disparities by relying on such technologies, given that mobile devices and health apps are most likely to be used by younger, educated women (Carroll et al., 2017).

Roberto also raised concern about precision nutrition being exploited for profit. She contended that food products are already exploited in this way, using the example of a fruit juice drink bearing multiple marketing messages, such as nutrient content claims, natural ingredient claims, and fruit and vegetable imagery. On the topic of profits, Roberto suggested that online shopping could be a positive or negative source of personalized marketing of foods. She noted that some retailers are already organizing their offerings by dietary preferences and using customers' browsing and purchasing data to recommend similar products, adding that this can be beneficial if the products are healthy foods but could exacerbate poor eating habits if the foods are unhealthy.

Roberto ended her remarks by referring to a framework for achieving health equity (Figure 4-1), which she proposed incorporating into the precision nutrition conversation. This framework, she explained, emphasizes the importance of developing interventions that aim to increase healthy options and/or reduce deterrents to unhealthy behaviors while also incorporating considerations related to social disadvantage and social determinants of health (Kumanyika, 2019). She appealed for "meeting people where they are" and pursuing strategies for making precision nutrition tools accessible for people with few resources.

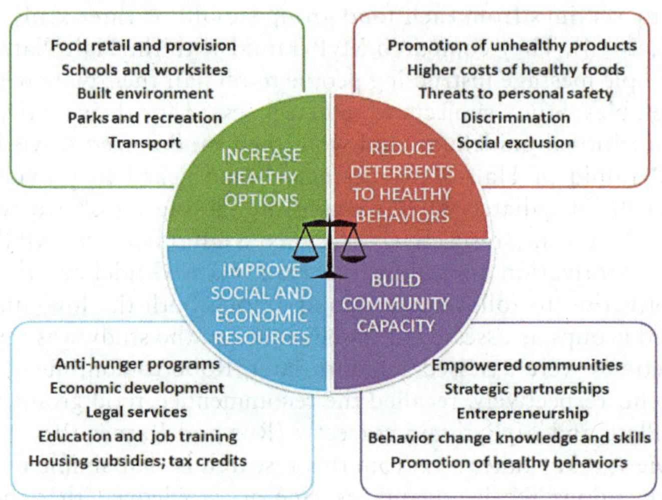

FIGURE 4-1 An equity-oriented obesity prevention action framework, which could be applied to precision nutrition efforts to assist in selecting or evaluating combinations of interventions that incorporate considerations related to social disadvantages and social determinants of health.
SOURCES: Presented by Christina Roberto on August 12, 2021; Kumanyika, 2017.

CHALLENGES TO IMPLEMENTING PRECISION NUTRITION

Peter Lurie, Center for Science in the Public Interest, prefaced his presentation by expressing excitement about the science underlying precision nutrition technologies, while cautioning that exciting science alone is not enough to improve public health. He argued that government has a role in supporting translation of the science into public health gains, but contended that current structures available to the government are inadequate to that task. Lurie supported this view by describing the history of precision medicine, whose promise, he stated, has been impeded for several decades. According to Lurie, some of that promise is finally being realized, but historically, the hype has exceeded what has been delivered.

Lurie suggested that one way to measure the increased focus on precision medicine at the FDA is by examining a category of products called companion diagnostics—diagnostic tests used as a companion to a therapeutic drug, biologic, or device. He noted that most FDA-approved companion diagnostic devices are for various cancers, and that these diagnostics can fall into a "regulatory vacuum" at the agency. He added that this is the case in particular for a subset of diagnostics called laboratory-developed tests (LDTs), a type of test for which the sample is collected in one location and submitted to another location for analysis.

According to Lurie, the FDA has exercised its enforcement authority over LDTs infrequently, in part because of industry assertions that they are subject to adequate oversight under the Comprehensive Laboratory Improvement Act (CLIA). But Lurie pointed out that the CLIA regulates laboratories, not tests, which he characterized as a problem that leads to a number of deficiencies in LDT oversight: a lack of evidence supporting the clinical validity of tests (i.e., how to use, interpret, and label a test and determine for whom it is indicated); inadequate adverse event reporting; lack of premarket review of performance data; unsupported manufacturer claims; inadequate product labeling because the focus is on the laboratory instead of the test; and an uneven playing field that he said results when some companies get premarket approval from the FDA and address these deficiencies while others do not. In 2020, the Secretary of Health and Human Services issued a memorandum stating that LDTs must be addressed individually in separate regulatory actions (to include *Federal Register* notices and comment periods), which Lurie maintained for practical purposes "is another way of saying there will be no regulation at all."

Lurie then gave three examples from what he said is a longer list of problematic LDTs, starting with an ovarian cancer screening test that detected a genetic variant thought to increase cancer risk and predict therapeutic response. A large independent study failed to confirm the variant's association with the suspected mutations, he recounted, meaning the test's detection of the variant's presence could effectively be a false positive that could lead to unnecessary surgery. A second problematic LDT, he continued, is a collection medium for the human papillomavirus test that is prone to false negatives for cancerous strains of the virus, presenting the risk of untreated cervical cancer. And a third example is an autism biomarker test that Lurie said lacks scientific basis but is used to develop a treatment plan for patients who screen positive (FDA, 2015).

Another complicating factor in FDA regulation, in Lurie's view, is its "general wellness" policy, stating that the agency does not intend to regulate general wellness products that (1) are intended to maintain or encourage a general state of health or healthy activity, and (2) present a low safety risk to users and other persons. Wellness products tend to fall into two categories, Lurie continued: those that do not make reference to treating, diagnosing, or preventing diseases or conditions (although such claims as "helps maintain a healthy weight" are permitted) and those that do not make reference to reducing risk of disease or helping people live with diseases or conditions unless the product is generally accepted as doing so (such as by tracking calories to reduce risk of type 2 diabetes). Many personalized nutrition offerings fall into these categories, he observed, making them exempt from premarket review of safety and adverse event reporting, and from having to prove that they follow good manufacturing processes, for example.

Lurie next described three types of claims about food that are permitted by FDA as another element of its regulation relevant to precision nutrition. First are health claims, which characterize the relationship between a substance and a disease and require "significant scientific agreement" and FDA preapproval before being used on food labels. Second are qualified health claims, which are similar but require a lower standard of evidence ("credible evidence"). Finally, structure/function claims describe a food's effect on the normal structure or function of the body and require "competent and reliable scientific evidence," as well as a disclaimer stating that the claim was not evaluated by FDA, and the product is not intended to diagnose, treat, cure, or prevent disease.

Lurie shared images of webpages for several personalized nutrition products that use these claims. Many appear to be structure/function claims, he observed, but he expressed doubt about the quality of the underlying evidence demonstrating support for and promotion of health. He cited as one example a test that measures one marker of immune response to nearly 100 foods, and suggests which foods to consider for an elimination diet. Whether that single marker of immune response is related to allergy and warrants avoiding certain foods is unsubstantiated, he asserted. Another example is a statement on a company's website that according to Lurie appeared to stray into health claim territory without apparent FDA approval. Lurie noted that FDA sends companies warning letters for food and supplement misbranding, and has sent more than 20 such letters each year for the past few years. If the agency had adequate resources, he contended, it would send many more such letters.

Lurie ended his presentation by appealing for better science and better regulation around precision nutrition. He argued that identifying a biological marker purported to be associated with increased risk of a disease is not equivalent to saying that intervening on that marker would have a measurable impact on a person's health, and that even if it were, intervention based on a personalized as opposed to a general approach would not necessarily make sound public health sense. The challenge is to identify when personalization versus a population-based approach makes most sense, he submitted, and he stressed that the choice between the two should be guided by which will have the most public health impact.

REGULATORY CHALLENGES AND OPPORTUNITIES
FOR PRECISION NUTRITION

Robert Califf, Verily and Google Health, provided a regulatory perspective on challenges and opportunities for precision nutrition, informed by his experience as FDA's deputy commissioner for medical products and tobacco (2015–2016) and commissioner of food and drugs (2016–2017).

FDA's mission is to preserve and protect the public health, he explained, making it a regulatory agency, a science agency, and a public health agency with the disciplines of science, medicine, public health, policy, and law simultaneously at play. He noted that the agency regulates human and veterinary drugs, biological products, medical devices, cosmetics, tobacco products, and radiation-emitting products, and asserted that the principles used to regulate those various products are often transferable to its regulation of food.

Although FDA is a science-based organization, Califf emphasized that it is also tasked with making decisions, even when more research would be helpful to clarify an optimal choice. He likened FDA's role to that of a referee making decisions with guidance from a rulebook, comprised of laws made by Congress, that it is responsible for interpreting and enforcing. The consequences of its actions are profound, he underscored, because the products it regulates represent about 20 percent of the U.S. economy and directly affect public health and patient well-being.

Califf discussed what he termed a "deteriorating" state of health among the U.S. public. The United States has the lowest life expectancy among the top 18 high-income countries worldwide (Ho and Hendi, 2018), he reported, and has lost even more ground on this metric in the wake of COVID-19, so that the gap in life expectancy between the United States and other high-income countries is now approaching 5 years (Woolf et al., 2021). The top 10 causes of death are dominated by chronic diseases, he added, with dietary factors being among the top risk factors driving death and disability (GBD 2019 Diseases and Injuries Collaborators, 2020).

Califf then highlighted a positive note in the context of the country's disappointing state of health—that the current data environment offers new capability to understand biology and behavior. As salient characteristics of the new data environment he cited real-time access to massive amounts of data, made possible by new methods of data storage; the ubiquity and liquidity of data; little to no delay in access to data; and the ability to analyze data rapidly to gain insights and develop guidance. Califf referenced the opportunity to intervene on a person's smartphone as an example of a capability that is a product of the new data environment and offers tremendous opportunity for providing precision nutrition guidance. The data-saturated environment enables integration of comprehensive health data, which he said is valuable both for assessing the entire human being and its interacting components and for generating evidence to inform public health decisions.

Califf's comment about the value of comprehensive health data led to his next point: that individual biomarkers are unlikely to predict a food's effect on health except in cases of specific nutritional deficiencies. He explained that for a biomarker of one measurement to serve as a surrogate (i.e., a substitute for a clinical endpoint), substantial evidence must exist to support that designation. The vast majority of biomarkers are not valid surrogates, he pointed out, because they exist in a milieu of biological complexity that provides many opportunities for error in predicting a health outcome. For this reason, he cautioned against making unsubstantiated claims that intermediate biomarkers will affect health in a predictable way. He referred attendees to the BEST (Biomarkers, EndpointS, and other Tools) Resource, a joint FDA–National Institutes of Health (NIH) project to develop a glossary of harmonized terminology for biomarkers and endpoints (FDA–NIH Biomarker Working Group, 2016).

In closing, Califf elaborated on the risk of intervening on surrogate endpoints represented by single biomarkers. He asserted that surrogates can be misleading by either overestimating or underestimating an intervention's effect on clinical outcomes (Fleming and DeMets, 1996), pointing out that an intervention can affect the biomarker of interest, the outcome of interest, or some other biological process in many unimagined ways. He expressed the hope that the emerging field of systems biology will provide unprecedented insights into the complex, multidimensional interplay of biological processes. According to Califf, the effect of food on health is a prime example of this complexity because many nutrients and substances interact simultaneously, each affecting multiple pathways and each with a potential impact on health. He added that biomarker tests—including those used for developing personalized nutrition guidance—need to be reliable and reproducible across multiple laboratories and clinical settings, and to maintain adequate sensitivity and specificity before the data they yield can be used in subsequent evaluation steps. Otherwise, he stressed, personalized recommendations could cause harm that might not be apparent until many years later.

LESSONS LEARNED ABOUT COMMERCIALIZING PERSONALIZED NUTRITION

Joshua Anthony, Nlumn,[2] shared lessons learned from his experience in the field. He began by observing that a variety of providers are rushing to understand how they can fit into the rapidly growing ecosystem of the personalized nutrition market (Figure 4-2), but they often make the mistake of putting themselves and their brand at the center when seeking to implement personalized nutrition. Instead, he said, it is critical to begin with consumers and examine their needs, behaviors, and values.

Anthony shared a series of insights about the profiles of people seeking personalized, food-based approaches to managing their health and wellness.

---

[2] Nlumn is a consulting company that works with food, nutrition, and health technology companies to help them compete in the personalized nutrition and health marketplace.

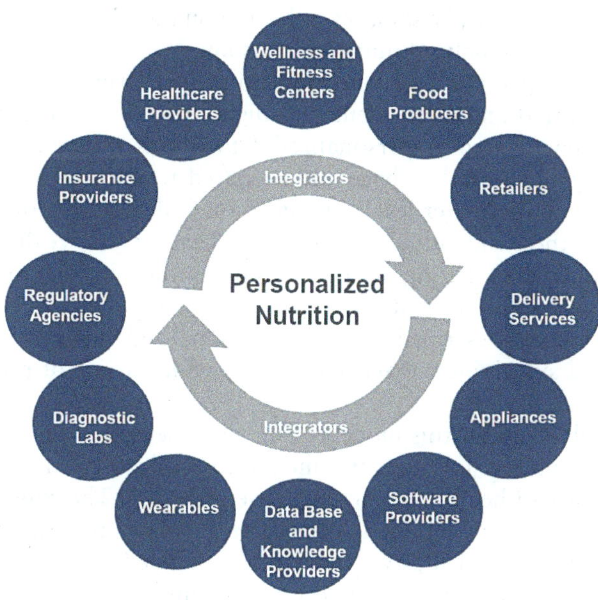

FIGURE 4-2 Various providers, tools, and services within the personalized nutrition ecosystem.
SOURCE: Presented by Joshua Anthony on August 12, 2021.

They hold widely different views about what health means, he noted, partly because of their different needs and partly because of their varying access to information or misinformation. Many people are turning away from experts and embracing scientific controversy, he observed, and seeking self-affirming information or groups aligned with their beliefs. He suggested the term "subjective personalization" to describe this behavior, which he said includes frequent shifting between different eating styles (e.g., ketogenic diet, intermittent fasting) to gain the different purported health benefits promised by each. A smaller proportion of consumers are seeking objective, data-driven personalization, Anthony continued. The challenge with this segment of consumers, he maintained, is that their expectations for the ability of online tools and wearables to help tailor their diet and behaviors are often ahead of the science supporting them, and very few providers have published results demonstrating improved health and functional outcomes.

Anthony described consumer expectations in the context of the current scientific landscape. Expectations for personalized nutrition's delivery of benefit solutions are broad and inconsistent, he asserted, ranging from managing chronic disease risk, to improving digestive health or joint pain, to maintaining sustained energy and reducing stress levels. Despite these differing expectations, he said, several common themes emerge in character-izing an ideal personalized nutrition consumer.

The ideal personalized nutrition consumer, Anthony continued, is highly motivated and goal oriented; a digitally savvy data tracker seeking objective advice based on personalized data who is willing and able to follow prescriptive lifestyle advice and prepared to manage and act on that information. With higher levels of education and socioeconomic status, he maintained, these individuals are relatively healthy and wealthy, highlighting the challenge of getting personalized nutrition solutions to populations of lower socioeconomic status.

Anthony next described a model of personalized nutrition that supports creating and sustaining engagement with a wide variety of potential users (Figure 4-3).

He explained that this model calls for first selecting the optimal health outcome of interest for the consumer, while collecting an objective, validated measure of health or function is the next step. The consumer's result for that measure, he continued, leads to personalized recommendations for improving health and lifestyle, which are intended to drive the behavior change necessary to achieve the desired outcome. The cyclical, continuous nature of the process supports engagement through reassessment and new advice, he added, as the consumer sets new outcome goals as health and functional needs change.

Anthony then described how providers can use the four aspects of the personalized nutrition engagement model to help design personalized nutrition offerings. When selecting a health outcome, he proposed focusing on a specific goal or benefit, which he said would allow solution providers to identify how their offerings can best deliver to fill one or more user need

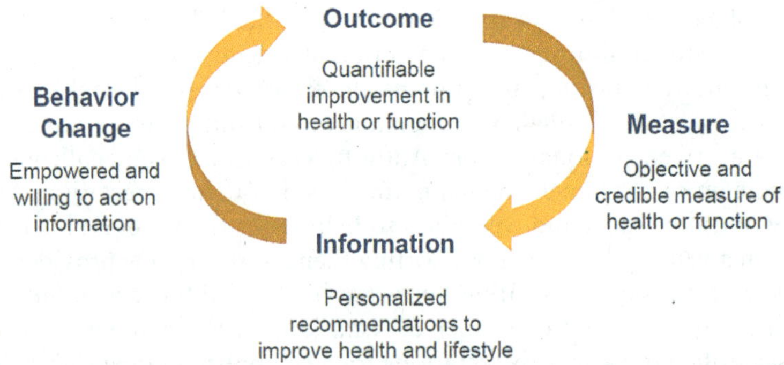

FIGURE 4-3 A model for personalized nutrition engagement.
SOURCES: Presented by Joshua Anthony on August 12, 2021; modified from Adams et al., 2020. Reprinted with permission from Oxford University Press.

gaps (gaps between desired user benefit and the current state). Anthony reiterated that user expectations are often ahead of the science, and that companies can differentiate their products and services by focusing on aspects of their program for which proof is provided by the existing evidence.

When assessing health or function, Anthony advised using validated diagnostic methods and measures (whether the metric is biological, behavioral, or sociological in nature); communicating instructions clearly to promote the collection of high-quality, accurate results; clarifying how the data will be used and how the measure is linked to a relevant benefit for the user's health; and being open to switching between validated diagnostic technologies to obtain a more robust assessment and avoid reliance on a specific technology that could become outdated.

Personalized recommendations based on a user's health assessment results will be more likely to drive behavior change, Anthony argued, if they are communicated consistent with the user's skill and experience. To enable behavior change, he continued, acknowledging and respecting user needs and preferences sets the tone for greater receptivity to objective suggestions for change. Small, frequent interactions offer opportunities to provide feedback and a reason to believe that change can be achieved, he observed, adding that the type and frequency of feedback are best personalized to the user. People still want a real person behind the technology, he maintained, noting that many programs use registered dietitians in this role as they can provide nutrition expertise and serve as behavior change mediators.

Anthony then discussed the state of the science of personalization. Companies can differentiate themselves by committing to evidence-based practices, he said, but most companies lack published data to support their program and its purported outputs. He added that companies may say that their program is supported by thousands of different studies, but usually this refers to research done by others. According to Anthony, personalized nutrition will be successful when it delivers health and functional benefits to users that go beyond one-size-fits-all approaches and are sustained over time (e.g., more than 12 months). In his view, most programs that are more rooted in science are just at the point where they are delivering or starting to show some health and functional benefits to users, but have yet to demonstrate that those benefits are sustainable and superior to outcomes from broader approaches.

Anthony concluded with three key takeaways for implementing personalized nutrition programs: identify a clear, compelling user-need gap to define the ideal consumer for the program instead of starting with the technology; build an engagement cycle around the ideal consumer and that person's user experience, so that users' inputs are commensurate with the outputs they receive; and continue to develop the program's proof points instead of relying solely on secondary sources for support.

COMMUNICATING THE BENEFITS OF PERSONALIZED
NUTRITION SOLUTIONS TO CONSUMERS

Martin Hahn, Hogan Lovells, U.S., LLP, discussed the future challenge of communicating the benefits of personalized nutrition solutions to the public while maintaining compliance with the current regulatory framework, which he said is not well designed to convey some of the industry's technological capabilities.

Hahn provided context for FDA's role in regulating food by explaining that it regulates products based on their intended use. Such use, he elaborated, determines whether a product is regulated as a drug or a dietary supplement, for example, and what types of claims it is permitted to carry. He briefly reiterated the various types of claims that products can bear, starting with disease claims for products intended to diagnosis, cure, mitigate, treat, or prevent disease. This type of claim will subject the product to regulation as an unapproved new drug or biologic, he explained, which he said is rational but can become complicated when the objective is to classify and communicate about nutritional interventions that purport to have a beneficial effect on disease. Echoing Lurie, he went on to say that health claims and qualified health claims are about reducing the risk of developing a disease, and structure/function claims are limited to the effect of the product on the body's structure or function.

Hahn pointed out what he called a paradox of structure/function claims—that many of them imply disease prevention. He provided examples of two approved structure/function claims—"calcium builds strong bones" and "whole oats support heart health"—implying reduced risk for osteoporosis and coronary heart disease, respectively. Despite support from competent, reliable scientific evidence, Hahn pointed out, these claims have the potential to convey a message that may not have been intended.

In Hahn's view, claims involve a tremendous tension between effectively conveying the intended message to consumers and remaining within regulatory guardrails. He identified as a related issue the need to ensure that statements made in advertising are both truthful and not misleading, which he explained is determined by the Federal Trade Commission (FTC). To make this determination, he said, FTC considers both explicit and implied messages conveyed by claims, meaning that companies are responsible for substantiating all reasonable interpretations of a claim with competent, reliable scientific evidence. For example, he elaborated, a cosmetic that is promoted as "age defying" may be supported by evidence that it increases skin elasticity, but if a certain threshold of consumers believe that the claim means the product will prevent wrinkles (when evidence does not exist to support this statement), the claim can be deemed false and misleading. This requirement creates further tension, he observed, in attempting to develop the short, pithy structure/function claims that many marketers insist are ideal for communicating to consumers.

Hahn next discussed challenges to communicating the benefits of personalized and precision nutrition. Communications must be truthful and not misleading, he emphasized, supported by competent, reliable scientific evidence for both explicit and reasonably implied claims. In Hahn's view, the evidence base for personalized nutrition is close to but not quite at the level needed to claim that certain types of diets will produce benefits for certain people with specific diseases and conditions. But, he stressed, when personalized nutrition technology reaches that point and communications about demonstrated health improvements are being developed for consumers, it will be important to have a regulatory structure that allows for communicating those benefits without unintended regulatory consequences.

Hahn then provided a series of examples to support his contention that the current regulatory system is not well suited to allowing the benefits of personalized nutrition technologies to be communicated without risking allegations of misleading consumers or being regulated in a way that is inconsistent with their intended use. As an example, he noted that a genetic analysis used to identify a diet that can help a healthy individual reduce the risk of developing diabetes could be communicated through an FDA-approved health claim, but if the genetic analysis is used to identify a diet that reduces insulin dependence for an individual with diagnosed diabetes, it is communicating a treatment effect and warrants a disease claim, which would trigger filing of the product as a drug. The new drug approval process is lengthy and expensive, he said, and could stifle innovation because it is not a viable option for many of the personalized nutrition technologies currently under way. A less risky structure/function claim could be made for a product, he added (e.g., that it supports blood glucose levels within normal ranges), but such a claim would not communicate the full benefits of the technology and likely would not attract as much consumer interest. In another example, he observed communicating a product's ability to alter the microbiome in a way that reduces the length and severity of the common cold would be making a disease claim, whereas making a structure/function claim such as "supports immune function" would be less risky but would not communicate in a clear, effective manner because it would underpromise the expected benefit.

Hahn urged stakeholder discussion toward developing a strategy for supporting a regulatory structure that would allow personalized nutrition technologies to advance and, when they have a sufficient evidence base, for clearly and effectively communicating their benefits to target populations without risking unintended regulatory consequences. Such a strategy, he posited could involve considering new legislation to give the FDA the authority to develop a new regulatory framework for personalized nutrition solutions, or adapting existing regulatory frameworks, such as those governing foods for special dietary uses or medical foods.

INCORPORATING PRECISION NUTRITION INTO FOOD-BASED AND NUTRIENT-BASED GUIDELINES

Patsy Brannon, Cornell University, discussed challenges and opportunities for incorporating precision nutrition into food- and nutrient-based guidelines for public health (such as the Dietary Reference Intakes [DRIs] and the *Dietary Guidelines for Americans* [USDA and HHS, 2020]), as well as into recommendations for individuals. She began by contrasting these two types of guidelines. Public health guidelines inform population-based policies and regulatory actions, such as federal nutrition programs, nutrition labeling, and population-level dietary intake assessments, she clarified, whereas individualized recommendations tailor nutrient and dietary intake, dietary patterns, and dietary intake assessment for a specific person. Public health guidelines are implemented through national outreach and education, policies and regulation, fortification, and population monitoring and assessment, she continued, which she acknowledged come with limitations resulting from their one-size-fits-all approach, but pointed out are necessary because it is not feasible to develop individualized recommendations for an entire population. Individualized recommendations are implemented through what Brannon called a "tech model" (an individual interacting with supported technology); a "hybrid model" (which adds a health professional to the supported technology); or a "self-directed model" (involving the individual's actions), which she suggested would entail individuals picking and choosing information from a variety of digital sources at the risk of taking in misinformation.

Public health guidelines must account for population-wide variation in individual needs, risks, preferences, and behaviors, Brannon observed, whereas individualized recommendations can be tailored to each of these aspects. She pointed out that moderate- to high-strength evidence is needed to support public health guidelines because of the risk to the population with lower levels of evidence quality. Turning to individualized recommendations, she suggested that they should be supported by at least moderate-strength evidence in either the tech model or hybrid model, but a lower level of evidence might be adequate for the self-directed model given the way individuals gather their information. Finally, she drew a distinction between public health guidelines, which are not directed at people with diseases that require medical nutrition therapy or that alter nutrition needs because of malabsorption, dialysis, disability, or altered mobility, and individualized recommendations, which may be able to include these individuals.

Brannon next reviewed the expanded DRI model, highlighting that it now includes the concept of chronic disease risk reduction (CDRR). She pointed out that chronic disease outcomes are no longer considered in determining either the estimated average requirement (EAR) or adequate intake for a nutrient, which are now based on an adequacy outcome, or the tolerable upper level (UL) for a nutrient, which is now based on toxicological outcomes. The notion of distribution of need is embedded in the expanded model, Brannon observed, noting that in a normal distribution of need, the EAR meets the needs of 50 percent of the population, while the recommended daily allowance (RDA) meets the needs of 97.5 percent of the population. She added, however, that an individual might have a need different from the RDA but still be included in the distribution of risk and need of the DRI framework.

Brannon explained that the formalization of chronic disease risk in the expanded DRI model can convey the potential for a variety of relationships to exist between such risk and dietary intake. To illustrate this point, she contrasted sodium, for which the risk of chronic disease increases as intake increases, and omega-3 fatty acids, for which the risk of chronic disease may decrease as intake increases. There could be other chronic diseases for which risk increases with intakes that are either too low or too high, she added, but in any case, the CDRR level is set to minimize chronic disease risk across the population.

Turning to the type of evidence needed to select adequacy and/or toxicity outcomes for a nutrient, Brannon explained that for adequacy, the indicator of nutrient status (i.e., biomarker) must be on the causal pathway to the clinical deficiency outcome of interest. Such outcomes relate to deficiency disorders, she elaborated, but the biomarkers can relate to effect (e.g., bone mineral density for calcium), exposure (e.g., red blood cell levels for folate), or mechanisms and functional outcomes (e.g., enzyme activity for thiamin). For adequacy and toxicity outcomes, respectively, the relationship between nutrient intake and the associated deficiency disorder or toxicologic effect must be supported by direct evidence. For adequacy, she continued, high certainty of causal and intake–response relationships is required (i.e., demonstrated by randomized controlled trials (RCTs), metabolic balance studies, or depletion/repletion studies).

Although the approach for setting DRI values requires examining the totality of the evidence using a rigorous, systematic review approach, Brannon pointed out that there are only 12 nutrients (total fat, omega-3 and omega-6 fatty acids, biotin, choline, vitamin K, pantothenic acid, chromium, fluoride, manganese, sodium, and potassium) for which the distribution of need is not yet understood, primarily because no adequacy outcome has been identified. Precision nutrition thus has an opportunity, she proposed, to help build stronger reference intake values for these nutrients as research leads to the identification of biomarkers of adequacy and their variance.

Brannon then clarified that DRIs for adequacy or toxicity are needed when the deficiency or toxicity of an essential nutrient is caused by that one nutrient, is prevented by nutritional interventions, and affects everyone if intake is inadequate or excessive. In contrast, she maintained, DRIs for CDRR purposes are not warranted without sufficient evidence of a relationship between the nutrient or a naturally occurring food substance and the risk of chronic disease. She added that such risk varies by individual, age, life stage, and various "omics," indicating the importance of systems biology approaches for understanding the relationships between chronic disease and nutrient intakes. Such relationships can be relative and/or small, she continued, are often related to many individual and environmental factors, and are only partly ameliorated by nutrition interventions. According to Brannon, precision nutrition has an opportunity to identify surrogate outcomes for chronic disease, even though having specific clinical disease outcomes is ideal (but difficult because discovering these outcomes requires longitudinal research).

Brannon also discussed the process for validating a surrogate outcome (i.e., intake of a nutrient, food, or dietary pattern) for chronic disease. First, the surrogate outcome must be on the causal pathway to disease, which she noted can be determined by observational and small interventional studies. Second, it must be concordant with changes in a health outcome that occur with a specific nutritional intervention, must be demonstrated in rigorous clinical trials, and must explain a clinically significant proportion of response to the nutritional intervention. Finally, it must accurately predict the effect of the nutritional intervention on the clinical outcome in rigorous clinical trials.

Brannon suggested that as precision nutrition advances, consideration be given to the evidence requirements for selecting chronic disease outcomes detailed in the *Guiding Principles for Developing Dietary Reference Intakes Based on Chronic Disease Outcomes* (NASEM, 2017) and applied by the DRI committee for sodium and potassium. She clarified that there must be at least moderate strength of evidence (based on GRADE [Grading of Recommendations Assessment, Development and Evaluation] methodology, a structured approach for evaluating the strength of evidence) for a causal association between the nutrient and a single specific chronic disease outcome or a single qualified surrogate outcome. She noted that the nature and substance of the evidence may vary from what is required to demonstrate adequacy, such that more evidence may come from observational studies than from RCTs, for example. Should that be the case, she said, there is lower certainty of a causal relationship because of the inherently greater risk of various types of bias with observational research.

Brannon next discussed an opportunity for precision nutrition to determine population subgroups with specific nutrient needs, including subgroups with distinctly different distributions of the requirement for a nutrient and response to its intake and subgroups of responders and non-responders to a nutrient. As an example of the latter, Brannon pointed out that the 2019 DRI committee for sodium and potassium noted the need to identify sodium-sensitive individuals through determination of "rare and common genetic variants" (NASEM, 2019). Subgroups may need to follow specific dietary patterns to mitigate risk of chronic disease, she continued, but evidence must be moderate to high for the causal association between dietary pattern and disease risk, as well as for the intake–response relationship. She identified as another opportunity for precision nutrition helping to fill the research gap of defining a "healthy population" when the prevalence of chronic disease is high. Doing so would promote better-informed public health guidelines for nutrients and dietary patterns, she argued, and enhance understanding of variance within a healthy population.

Brannon next raised the issue of whether individual algorithms can be linked to public health guidelines. She observed that a major challenge in both clinical and dietetics practice is the difficulty of confirming an individual's specific nutrient requirements, although she stressed that this challenge does not invalidate the typical public health population approach of basing recommendations on a normal distribution of nutrient requirements. At the same time, she said, differences in individual needs could create opportunities for both adequacy and chronic disease DRIs and for the *Dietary Guidelines* (USDA and HHS, 2020) to be more tailored to individuals, although the strength of evidence required for such tailoring remains to be determined.

Brannon pointed out that individual guidelines based on precision nutrition also raise the issue of efficacy versus effectiveness. She affirmed that some precision nutrition approaches have demonstrated efficacy, but suggested that the effectiveness of these findings may be subject to bias due to self-selection of participants. She encouraged consideration of theories of behavior change—such as the health belief model, theory of planned behavior, transtheoretical model (stages of change), and precaution adoption process model—that could provide insight into characteristics of participants, such as perceptions of health risks and of avoiding those risks, perceived control over one's health, and degree of motivation and readiness to change.

To end her presentation, Brannon highlighted four questions. First, how can we develop blended models that address the needs for both population food- and nutrient-based guidelines and individualized precision nutrition recommendations? Second, what is an effective strategy for communicating both types of guidelines? Third, how do we ensure equitable access for people at highest risk of poor health (e.g., individuals with low incomes, lack of health insurance, food insecurity, lack of housing, low health literacy)? And fourth, how do we ensure that practitioners receive an appropriate scope and depth of training to implement individual guidelines?

PANEL DISCUSSION

Health Claims for Targeted Populations

An audience member observed that existing FDA-approved nutrition-related health claims apply to the general population, and asked whether health claims for precision nutrition interventions would require claims for targeted populations. Califf said he did not see a reason for the FDA to allow a product to carry a health claim for the general population with respect to a benefit that applies only to a targeted population. Lurie agreed that a health claim should not exceed the evidence supporting it. He added that practically speaking, companies might not want to make restricted claims because doing so would limit the target audience for their products. Hahn contended that not allowing a claim for a targeted population would represent a missed opportunity, and suggested that designated medical foods (which are designed to address an individual's unique needs resulting from a disease) could carry these types of claims. Lurie countered that the medical foods pathway is unattractive from a commercialization point of view because it requires a physician intermediary.

Preventing Erosion of Public Trust in Precision and Personalized Nutrition Solutions

An audience member alluded to the erosion of consumer trust in public health guidance during the COVID-19 pandemic and asked how to avoid the same response to personalized nutrition solutions. Califf underscored the importance of maintaining scientific integrity in messages aimed at connecting emotionally with consumers to effect behavior change. Anthony appealed for building trust and transparency with consumers by being honest about the strengths and limitations of a personalized nutrition solution. Brannon alluded to the challenge of communicating to the public about evolving science and public health topics when guidance may change as additional evidence becomes available. Lurie agreed and added that the pace of evolution in scientific understanding is not commensurate with the pace of new claims circulating through the Internet, and that the regulatory process for policing claims and bringing enforcement action against false claims is quite slow.

Incorporating Social Determinants of Health in Precision and Personalized Nutrition Models

Brannon agreed with an audience member's comment that it is important to incorporate social determinants of health into precision nutrition models, and suggested that also incorporating constructs from behavior change theory can help predict consumer success with uptake of recommendations. For example, asking people about their perceived barriers to change can inform how they will respond to personalized nutrition guidance. Roberto agreed that incorporating social determinants of health is critical for ensuring that people receive recommendations that are not only matched to their biological attributes but also actionable in their cultural, community, and economic contexts. Califf pointed out that behavioral attributes are just as measurable as biological attributes, and that a common practice in advertising is to segment populations by behavioral phenotypes. He warned that if a product's profit is higher in one population segment than another, it introduces risk that the unprofitable segment may not be included in research unless a requirement for inclusive research designs exists.

N-of-1 Study Designs

In response to an audience member's question about the role of n-of-1 study designs in personalized nutrition, Califf replied that n-of-1 is a great design when the objective is to assess an intervention's short-term effects in an individual. He noted, however, that a primary risk with this design is drawing incorrect conclusions because short-term changes in a biomarker are often not predictive of the overall long-term outcome. In Lurie's view, n-of-1 designs are most useful when the mechanism of action is clearly defined and outcome measures are objective. Anthony suggested that the strongest evidence from n-of-1 study designs comes from crossover studies, and Califf contended that subjective outcomes are appropriate in n-of-1 studies if a crossover design with a placebo is used. Roberto advocated for studying broad groups in any research design that is used, pointing out that if at baseline, more narrowly defined study populations are already healthier than groups not included in the study, relationships will look stronger for any positive health effects observed in response to the nutrition intervention being studied.

Developing Blended Models to Address Population and Individual Needs

Brannon speculated as to whether public health models could provide general recommendations while also stating that additional guidance for tailoring certain recommendations was available for people with specific characteristics. This approach would apply in the case of sodium, she said in reference to Hilliard's presentation earlier in the workshop, for which a subset of the African American population had much lower needs relative to other population groups.

Anthony suggested that "personalized nutrition" is the term that will best resonate with consumers, whereas "precision nutrition" may be construed as narrowly focused on measurement of biomarkers hitting specific targets for nutrient intake. He suggested that the latter is unnecessarily prescriptive and does not account for the personal preferences, beliefs, and values that influence an individual's food choices.

Applying Personalized Nutrition to Family Meals

An audience member asked the speakers how they envision implementation of personalized nutrition at the family level, when each family member may have different food plans. Lurie responded that a great deal of work would be required to customize meals for each family member, and suggested that increased precision could also increase complexity and confusion. He noted that people sometimes accept degrees of imprecision because such messaging is simpler, and proposed that increased precision in nutrition guidance is not necessarily worth the potential risk of increased confusion until stronger data are available to support the associated health benefits. Califf added that food access and availability influence the degree to which people are able to follow specific dietary guidance. Roberto suggested that it would be helpful to have pre-prepared, good-tasting, convenient meal solutions for people who do not always have time to prepare customized meals for their families. Brannon pointed out that when certain family members have special dietary needs, the family often chooses meals with components that can easily be adapted for those needs. These families would likely find it helpful to work with a registered dietitian or other expert, she proposed, so they could learn how to translate special dietary needs into food choices and recipes. And according to Anthony, one family member's special dietary needs or preferences can encourage food exploration by other family members.

Personalized Nutrition's Potential to Improve Food Access

Hahn speculated whether personalized nutrition recommendations could promote increased access to healthy foods in underserved communities. Lurie pointed out that in the pharmaceutical market, drugs developed for targeted populations are sold at a higher price point relative to drugs for broader populations. People are willing to pay more for something they believe is tailored to their specific needs, he proposed, but added that higher prices also restrict access to those products. Califf noted that certain grocery stores are intentionally located in higher-income areas and suggested that greater transparency about retailer siting could lead people to demand more equitable distribution of retail food venues. Brannon cautioned against the use of unnecessarily restrictive messaging that leads people to believe, for example, that they must choose fresh forms of fruits and vegetables. Minimally processed canned and frozen produce is as nutritious as fresh varieties, she pointed out, and its affordability and shelf stability make it more accessible for people with limited resources. To clarify, she added that more flexible guidance helps people make choices that address the various factors they must weigh when making food choices. Anthony suggested that increased personalization may increase food waste, but the foods that do not meet one group's personalized plans could be minimally processed into other foods that meet another group's needs (rather than being discarded). Although this approach could help improve food access, he cautioned that it could result in the appearance that one population is getting "seconds."

Exciting Aspects of Precision and Personalized Nutrition

Before concluding the panel discussion, McKinnon invited the six speakers to share aspects of the precision and personalized nutrition field that are particularly exciting to them. Hahn responded that the science is advancing to the point of being actionable. The science is fascinating, Roberto agreed, and added that it is spurring conversations about related environmental, political, economic, and social issues that are introduced by precision and personalized nutrition opportunities. Lurie echoed Roberto's thoughts and added that he was encouraged to be discussing these issues while the technology is still emerging, rather than having to manage misinformation and unintended consequences down the road. Califf expressed excitement about the opportunities to measure behavioral and environmental factors and their interactions, and Anthony highlighted the potential to combine those measures with biological measures in a systems approach that can make personal nutrition solutions more widely accessible. Finally, Brannon voiced hope for the prospect of translating the effective aspects of personalized nutrition platforms into innovative solutions for implementing public health guidelines.

References

Acosta, A., M. Camilleri, A. Shin, M. I. Vazquez-Roque, J. Iturrino, D. Burton, J. O'Neill, D. Eckert, and A. R. Zinsmeister. 2015. Quantitative gastrointestinal and psychological traits associated with obesity and response to weight-loss therapy. *Gastroenterology* 148(3):537–546.e4.

Acosta A., M. Camilleri, B. Abu Dayyeh, G. Calderon, D. Gonzalez, A. McRae, W. Rossini, S. Singh, D. Burton, and M. M. Clark. 2021. Selection of antiobesity medications based on phenotypes enhances weight loss: A pragmatic trial in an obesity clinic. *Obesity (Silver Spring)* 29(4):662–671.

Adams, S. H., J. C. Anthony, R. Carvajal, L. Chae, C. Khoo, M. E. Latulippe, N. V. Matusheski, H. L. McClung, M. Rozga, C. H. Schmid, S. Wopereis, and W. Yan. 2020. Perspective: Guiding principles for the implementation of personalized nutrition approaches that benefit health and function. *Advances in Nutrition (Bethesda)* 11(1):25–34.

Adhikari, A. N., R. C. Gallagher, Y. Wang, R. J. Currier, G. Amatuni, L. Bassaganyas, F. Chen, K. Kundu, M. Kvale, S. D. Mooney, R. L. Nussbaum, S. S. Randi, J. Sanford, J. T. Shieh, R. Srinivasan, U. Sunderam, H. Tang, D. Vaka, Y. Zou, B. A. Koenig, P-Y. Kwok, N. Risch, J. M. Puck, and S. E. Brenner. 2020a. The role of exome sequencing in newborn screening for inborn errors of metabolism. *Nature Medicine* 26(9):1392–1397.

Adhikari, S., E. C. Nice, E. W. Deutsch, L. Lane, G. S. Omenn, S. R. Pennington, Y.-K. Paik, C. M. Overall, F. J. Corrales, I. M. Cristea, J. E. Van Eyk, M. Uhlén, C. Lindskog, D. W. Chan, A. Bairoch, J. C. Waddington, J. L. Justice, J. LaBaer, H. Rodriguez, F. He, M. Kostrzewa, P. Ping, R. L. Gundry, P. Stewart, S. Srivastava, S. Srivastava, F. C. S. Nogueira, G. B. Domont, Y. Vandenbrouck, M. P. Y. Lam, S. Wennersten, J. A. Vizcaino, M. Wilkins, J. M. Schwenk, E. Lundberg, N. Bandeira, G. Marko-Varga, S. T. Weintraub, C. Pineau, U. Kusebauch, R. L. Moritz, S. B. Ahn, M. Palmblad, M. P. Snyder, R. Aebersold, and M. S. Baker. 2020b. A high-stringency blueprint of the human proteome. *Nature Communications* 11(1).

Antonio, J., S. Knafo, M. Kenyon, A. Ali, C. Carson, A. Ellerbroek, C. Weaver, J. Roberts, C. A. Peacock, and J. L. Tartar. 2019. Assessment of the FTO gene polymorphisms (rs1421085, rs17817449 and rs9939609) in exercise-trained men and women: The effects of a 4-week hypocaloric diet. *Journal of the International Society of Sports Nutrition* 16.

Aral, S., and C. Nicolaides. 2017. Exercise contagion in a global social network. *Nature Communications* 8.

Bassolas, A., H. Barbosa-Filho, B. Dickinson, X. Dotiwalla, P. Eastham, R. Gallotti, G. Ghoshal, B. Gipson, S. A. Hazarie, H. Kautz, O. Kucuktunc, A. Lieber, A. Sadilek, and J. J. Ramasco. 2019. Hierarchical organization of urban mobility and its connection with city livability. *Nature Communications* 10(4817).

Ben-Yacov, O., A. Godneva, M. Rein, S. Shilo, D. Kolobkov, N. Koren, N. Cohen Dolev, T. Travinsky Shmul, B. C. Wolf, N. Kosower, K. Sagiv, M. Lotan-Pompan, N. Zmora, A. Weinberger, E. Elinav, and E. Segal. 2021. Personalized postprandial glucose response-targeting diet versus Mediterranean diet for glycemic control in prediabetes. *Diabetes Care* 44(9):1980–1991.

Berry, S. E., A. M. Valdes, D. A. Drew, F. Asnicar, M. Mazidi, J. Wolf, J. Capdevila, G. Hadjigeorgiou, R. Davies, H. Al Khatib, C. Bonnett, S. Ganesh, E. Bakker, D. Hart, M. Mangino, J. Merino, I. Linenberg, P. Wyatt, J. M. Ordovas, C. D. Gardner, et al. 2020. Human postprandial responses to food and potential for precision nutrition. *Nature Medicine* 26(6):964–973.

Boutelle, K. N., D. E. Kang Sim, M. Manzano, K. E. Rhee, S. J. Crow, and D. R. Strong. 2019. Role of appetitive phenotype trajectory groups on child body weight during a family-based treatment for children with overweight or obesity. *International Journal of Obesity* 43(11):2302–2308.

Boutelle, K. N., M. A. Manzano, and D. M. Eichen. 2020. Appetitive traits as targets for weight loss: The role of food cue responsiveness and satiety responsiveness. *Physiology & Behavior* 224:113018.

Carnell, S., and J. Wardle. 2008. Appetite and adiposity in children: Evidence for a behavioral susceptibility theory of obesity. *American Journal of Clinical Nutrition* 88(1):22–29.

Carnell, S., C. M. Haworth, R. Plomin, and J. Wardle. 2008. Genetic influence on appetite in children. *International Journal of Obesity* 32(10):1468–1473.

Carnell, S., K. Pryor, L. A. Mais, S. Warkentin, L. Benson, and R. Cheng. 2016. Lunch-time food choices in preschoolers: Relationships between absolute and relative intakes of different food categories, and appetitive characteristics and weight. *Physiology & Behavior* 162:151–160.

Carroll, J. K., A. Moorhead, R. Bond, W. G. LeBlanc, R. J. Petrella, and K. Fiscella. 2017. Who uses mobile phone health apps and does use matter? A secondary data analytics approach. *Journal of Medical Internet Research* 19(4):e125.

Celis-Morales, C., K. M. Livingstone, C. F. Marsaux, A. L. Macready, R. Fallaize, C. B. O'Donovan, C. Woolhead, H. Forster, M. C. Walsh, S. Navas-Carretero, R. San-Cristobal, L. Tsirigoti, C. P. Lambrinou, C. Mavrogianni, G. Moschonis, S. Kolossa, J. Hallmann, M. Godlewska, A. Surwillo, I. Traczyk, et al. 2017. Effect of personalized nutrition on health-related behaviour change: Evidence from the Food4Me European randomized controlled trial. *International Journal of Epidemiology* 46(2):578–588.

Centola, D. 2011. An experimental study of homophily in the adoption of health behavior. *Science* 336(6060):1269–1272.

Chao, A. M., T. A. Wadden, A. A. Gorin, J. Shaw Tronieri, R. L. Pearl, Z. M. Bakizada, S. Z. Yanovski, and R. I. Berkowitz. 2017. Binge eating and weight loss outcomes in individuals with type 2 diabetes: 4-year results from the Look AHEAD Study. *Obesity (Silver Spring)* 25(11):1830–1837.

Chetty, R., M. Stepner, S. Abraham, S. Lin, B. Scuderi, N. Turner, A. Bergeron, and D. Cutler. 2016. The association between income and life expectancy in the United States, 2001-2014. *JAMA* 315(16):1750–1766.

de la Haye, K., G. Robins, P. Mohr, and C. Wilson. 2011. Homophily and contagion as explanations for weight similarities among adolescent friends. *The Journal of Adolescent Health* 49(4):421–427.

de La Haye, K., G. Robins, P. Mohr, and C. Wilson. 2013. Adolescents' intake of junk food: Processes and mechanisms driving consumption similarities among friends. *Journal of Research on Adolescence* 23(3):524–536.

de Luis, D. A., R. Aller, O. Izaola, D. Primo, S. Urdiales, and E. Romero. 2015. Effects of a high-protein/low-carbohydrate diet versus a standard hypocaloric diet on weight and cardiovascular risk factors: Role of a genetic variation in the rs9939609 FTO gene variant. *Journal of Nutrigenetics and Nutrigenomics* 8(3):128–136.

Delormier, T., K. L. Frohlich, and L. Potvin. 2009. Food and eating as social practice—understanding eating patterns as social phenomena and implications for public health. *Sociology of Health & Illness* 31(2):215–228.

FDA (Food and Drug Administration). 2015. *The public health evidence or FDA oversight of laboratory developed tests: 20 case studies.* Washington, DC: Food and Drug Administration. https://wayback.archive-it.org/7993/20171115144712/https://www.fda.gov/downloads/AboutFDA/ReportsManualsForms/Reports/UCM472777.pdf (accessed October 11, 2021).

FDA–NIH (National Institutes of Health) Biomarker Working Group. 2016. *BEST (Biomarkers, EndpointS, and other Tools) Resource.* Silver Spring, MD: U.S. Food and Drug Administration. https://www.ncbi.nlm.nih.gov/books/NBK326791/pdf/Bookshelf_NBK326791.pdf (accessed October 11, 2021).

Fildes, A., K. M. Mallan, L. Cooke, C. H. M. van Jaarsveld, C. H. Llewellyn, A. Fisher, and L. Daniels. 2015. The relationship between appetite and food preferences in British and Australian children. *International Journal of Behavioral Nutrition and Physical Activity* 12(116).

Fleming, T. R., and D. L. DeMets. 1996. Surrogate end points in clinical trials: Are we being misled? *Annals of Internal Medicine* 125(7):605–613.

Fletcher, A., C. Bonell, and A. Sorhaindo. 2011. You are what your friends eat: Systematic review of social network analyses of young people's eating behaviours and bodyweight. *Journal of Epidemiology and Community Health* 65:548–555.

Fuzo, C. A., U. da Veiga, S. Moco, O. Cominetti, S. Métairon, S. Pruvost, A. Charpagne, J. Carayol, R. Torrieri, W. A. Silva Jr, P. Descombes, J. Kaput, and J. P. Monteiro. 2021. Contribution of genetic ancestry and polygenic risk score in meeting vitamin B12 needs in healthy Brazilian children and adolescents. *Scientific Reports* 11(1).

Garcia-Bailo, B., and A. El-Sohemy. 2021. Recent advances and current controversies in genetic testing for personalized nutrition. *Current Opinion in Clinical Nutrition and Metabolic Care* 24(4):289–295.

Gardner, C. D., J. F. Trepanowski, L. C. Del Gobbo, M. E. Hauser, J. Rigdon, J. P. A. Ioannidis, M. Desai, and A. C. King. 2018. Effect of low-fat vs low-carbohydrate diet on 12-month weight loss in overweight adults and the association with genotype pattern or insulin secretion: The DIETFITS randomized clinical trial. *Journal of the American Medical Association* 319(7):667–679.

GBD (Global Burden of Disease) 2019 Diseases and Injuries Collaborators. 2020. Global burden of 369 diseases and injuries in 204 countries and territories, 1990-2019: A systematic analysis for the Global Burden of Disease Study 2019. *Lancet* 396(10258):1204–1222.

Ho, J. Y., and A. S. Hendi. 2018. Recent trends in life expectancy across high income countries: Retrospective observational study. *British Medical Journal* 362:k3622.

Homann, C. M., C. A. J. Rossel, S. Dizzell, L. Bervoets, J. Simioni, J. Li, E. Gunn, M. G. Surette, R. J. de Souza, M. Mommers, E. K. Hutton, K. M. Morrison, J. Penders, N. van Best, and J. C. Stearns. 2021. Infants' first solid foods: Impact on gut microbiota development in two intercontinental cohorts. *Nutrients* 3(8):2639.

Horne, J., J. Gilliland, C. O'Connor, J. Seabrook, and J. Madill. 2020. Enhanced long-term dietary change and adherence in a nutrigenomics-guided lifestyle intervention compared to a population-based (GLB/DPP) lifestyle intervention for weight management: Results from the NOW randomised controlled trial. *BMJ Nutrition, Prevention & Health* 3(1):49–59.

Hudson, J. I., E. Hiripi, H. G. Pope Jr, and R. C. Kessler. 2007. The prevalence and correlates of eating disorders in the National Comorbidity Survey Replication. *Biological Psychiatry* 61(3):348–358.

Hunot, C., A. Fildes, H. Croker, C. H. Llewellyn, J. Wardle, and R. J. Beeken. 2016. Appetitive traits and relationships with BMI in adults: Development of the Adult Eating Behaviour Questionnaire. *Appetite* 105:356–363.

Jinnette, R., A. Narita, B. Manning, S. A. McNaughton, J. C. Mathers, and K. M. Livingstone. 2021. Does personalized nutrition advice improve dietary intake in healthy adults? A systematic review of randomized controlled trials. *Advances in Nutrition (Bethesda)* 12(3):657–669.

Johnson, A. J., P. Vangay, G. A. Al-Ghalith, B. M. Hillmann, T. L. Ward, R. R. Shields-Cutler, A. D. Kim, A. K. Shmagel, A. N. Syed, Personalized Microbiome Class Students, J. Walter, R. Menon, K. Koecher, and D. Knights. 2019. Daily sampling reveals personalized diet-microbiome associations in humans. *Cell Host & Microbe* 25(6):789–802.e5.

Johnson, A. J., J. J. Zheng, J. W. Kang, A. Saboe, D. Knights, and A. M. Zivkovic. 2020. A guide to diet-microbiome study design. *Frontiers in Nutrition* 7:79.

Kahneman, D. 2003. Maps of bounded rationality: Psychology for behavioral economics. *The American Economic Review* 93(5):1449–1475.

Kaplan, L. M. 2017. *Treating obesity: A 2017 overview* [Conference presentation]. Harvard Blackburn Course in Obesity Medicine: Treating Obesity 2017, Boston, MA.

Kininmoth, A. R., A. D. Smith, C. H. Llewellyn, and A. Fildes. 2020. Socioeconomic status and changes in appetite from toddlerhood to early childhood. *Appetite* 146.

Koehly, L. M., and A. Loscalzo. 2009. Adolescent obesity and social networks. *Preventing Chronic Disease* 6(3):A99.

Kumanyika, S. K. 2017. Getting to equity in obesity prevention: A new framework. *NAM Perspectives*. Discussion Paper. Washington, DC: National Academy of Medicine.

Kumanyika, S. K. 2019. A framework for increasing equity impact in obesity prevention. *American Journal of Public Health* 109:1350–1357.

Lewis, C. E., K. M. McTigue, L. E. Burke, P. Poirier, R. H. Eckel, B. V. Howard, D. B. Allison, S. Kumanyika, and F. X. Pi-Sunyer. 2009. Mortality, health outcomes, and body mass index in the overweight range: A science advisory from the American Heart Association. *Circulation* 119(25):3263–3271.

Lonardo, A., A. Mantovani, S. Lugari, and G. Targher. 2020. Epidemiology and pathophysiology of the association between NAFLD and metabolically healthy or metabolically unhealthy obesity. *Annals of Hepatology* 19(4):359–366.

Llewellyn, C. H., C. H. van Jaarsveld, L. Johnson, S. Carnell, and J. Wardle. 2010. Nature and nurture in infant appetite: Analysis of the Gemini twin birth cohort. *American Journal of Clinical Nutrition* 91(5):1172–1179.

Llewellyn, C. H., C. H. van Jaarsveld, L. Johnson, S. Carnell, and J. Wardle. 2011. Development and factor structure of the Baby Eating Behaviour Questionnaire in the Gemini birth cohort. *Appetite* 57(2):388–396.

Madden, J., C. M. Williams, P. C. Calder, G. Lietz, E. A. Miles, H. Cordell, J. C. Mathers, A. M. Minihane. 2011. The impact of common gene variants on the response of biomarkers of cardiovascular disease (CVD) risk to increased fish oil fatty acids intakes. *Annual Review of Nutrition* 31:203–234.

Mathias, M. G., C. A. Coelho-Landell, M. P. Scott-Boyer, S. Lacroix, M. J. Morine, R. G. Salomão, R. Toffano, M. Almada, J. M. Camarneiro, E. Hillesheim, T. T. de Barros, J. S. Camelo-Junior, E. Campos Giménez, K. Redeuil, A. Goyon, E. Bertschy, A. Lévêques, J. M. Oberson, C. Giménez, J. Carayol, et al. 2018. Clinical and vitamin response to a short-term multi-micronutrient intervention in Brazilian children and teens: From population data to interindividual responses. *Molecular Nutrition & Food Research* 62(6):e1700613.

McPherson, M., L. Smith-Lovin, and J. M. Cook. 2001. Birds of a feather: Homophily in social networks. *Annual Review of Sociology* 27(1):415–444.

Merritt, D. C., J. Jamnik, and A. El-Sohemy. 2018. FTO genotype, dietary protein intake, and body weight in a multiethnic population of young adults: A cross-sectional study. *Genes & Nutrition* 13.

Mirtchouk, M., D. L. McGuire, A. L. Deierlein, and S. Kleinberg. 2019. Automated estimation of food type from body-worn audio and motion sensors in free-living environments. *Proceedings of Machine Learning Research* 106:641–662.

Mooreville, M., A. Davey, A. Orloski, E. L. Hannah, K. C. Mathias, L. L. Birch, T. V. Kral, I. F. Zakeri, and J. O. Fisher. 2015. Individual differences in susceptibility to large portion sizes among obese and normal-weight children. *Obesity* 23(4):808–814.

NASEM (National Academies of Sciences, Engineering, and Medicine). 2017. *Guiding principles for developing dietary reference intakes based on chronic disease.* Washington, DC: The National Academies Press.

NASEM. 2019. *Dietary reference intakes for sodium and potassium.* Washington, DC: The National Academies Press.

NHGRI (National Human Genome Research Institute). 2020. *Epigenomics fact sheet.* Bethesda, MD: National Institutes of Health. https://www.genome.gov/about-genomics/fact-sheets/Epigenomics-Fact-Sheet (accessed October 11, 2021).

NHS (National Health Service) Digital. 2014. *National Child Measurement Programme: England, 2013/14 school year.* https://digital.nhs.uk/data-and-information/publications/statistical/national-child-measurement-programme/2013-14-school-year (accessed October 11, 2021).

Nielsen, D. E., and A. El-Sohemy. 2014. Disclosure of genetic information and change in dietary intake: A randomized controlled trial. *PloS One* 9(11):e112665.

NIH (National Institutes of Health). 2017. *Story of discovery—APOL1 gene variants: Unraveling the genetic basis of elevated risk for kidney disease in African Americans.* Washington, DC: National Institute of Diabetes and Digestive and Kidney Diseases. https://www.niddk.nih.gov/news/archive/2017/story-variants-unraveling-genetic-basis-elevated-risk-kidney-disease-african-americans (accessed September 27, 2021).

Ordovas, J. M., L. R. Ferguson, E. S. Tai, and J. C. Mathers. 2018. Personalised nutrition and health. *British Medical Journal* 361:bmj.k2173.

Ratner, R. K., and J. Riis. 2014. Communicating science-based recommendations with memorable and actionable guidelines. *Proceedings of the National Academy of Sciences* 111(Suppl 4):13634–13641.

Riis, J., and R. K. Ratner. 2011. Simplified nutrition guidelines to fight obesity. In R. Batra, P. A. Keller, V. J. Strecher (Eds.). *Leveraging consumer psychology for effective health communications: The obesity challenge.* Armonk, NY: Routledge.

Roberto, C. A., B. Swinburn, C. Hawkes, T. T. Huang, S. A. Costa, M. Ashe, L. Zwicker, J. H. Cawley, and K. D. Brownell. 2015. Patchy progress on obesity prevention: Emerging examples, entrenched barriers, and new thinking. *Lancet* 385(9985):2400–2409.

Rodgers, G. P., and F. S. Collins. 2020. Precision nutrition—the answer to "What to eat to stay healthy." *Journal of the American Medical Association* 324(8):735–736.

Rodriguez, L. R., E. B. Rasmussen, D. Kyne-Rucker, M. Wong, and K. S. Martin. 2021. Delay discounting and obesity in food insecure and food secure women. *Health Psychology* 40(4):242–251.

Schüssler-Fiorenza Rose, S. M., K. Contrepois, K. J. Moneghetti, W. Zhou, T. Mishra, S. Mataraso, O. Dagan-Rosenfeld, A. B. Ganz, J. Dunn, D. Hornburg, S. Rego, D. Perelman, S. Ahadi, M. R. Sailani, Y. Zhou, S. R. Leopold, J. Chen, M. Ashland, J. W. Christle, M. Avina, P. Limcaoco, C. Ruiz, M. Tan, A. J. Butte, G. M. Weinstock, G. M. Slavich, E. Sodergren, T. L. McLaughlin, F. Haddad, and M. P. Snyder. 2019. A longitudinal big data approach for precision health. *Nature Medicine* 25(5):792–804.

Smith, K. R., E. Jansen, G. Thapaliya, A. H. Aghababian, L. Chen, J. R. Sadler, and S. Carnell. 2021. The influence of COVID-19-related stress on food motivation. *Appetite* 163:105233.

Taberlet, P., E. Coissac, F. Pompanon, C. Brochmann, and E. Willerslev. 2012. Towards next-generation biodiversity assessment using DNA metabarcoding. *Molecular Ecology* 21(8):2045–2050.

Tanofsky-Kraff, M., N. A. Schvey, and C. M. Grilo. 2020. A developmental framework of binge-eating disorder based on pediatric loss of control eating. *The American Psychologist* 75(2):189–203.

Thomas, D. M., B. Siegel, D. Baller, J. Lindquist, G. Cready, J. T. Zervios, J. F. Nadglowski Jr, and T. K. Kyle. 2020. Can the participant speak beyond Likert? Free-text responses in COVID-19 obesity surveys. *Obesity* 28(12):2268–2271.

Trogdon, J. G., J. Nonnemaker, and J. Pais. 2008. Peer effects in adolescent overweight. *Journal of Health Economics* 27(5):1388–1399.

Turnwald, B. P., J. P. Goyer, D. Z. Boles, A. Silder, S. L. Delp, and A. J. Crum. 2019. Learning one's genetic risk changes physiology independent of actual genetic risk. *Nature Human Behaviour* 3:48–56.

USDA (U.S. Department of Agriculture) and Agricultural Research Service. 2020. Nutrient intakes from food and beverages: Mean amounts consumed per individual, by gender and age. *What We Eat in America, NHANES 2017-2018.* https://www.ars.usda.gov/ARSUserFiles/80400530/pdf/1718/Table_1_NIN_GEN_17.pdf (accessed October 11, 2021).

USDA and HHS (U.S. Department of Health and Human Services). 2020. *Dietary Guidelines for Americans, 2020-2025.* Washington, DC: U.S. Department of Agriculture. https://www.dietaryguidelines.gov/sites/default/files/2021-03/Dietary_Guidelines_for_Americans-2020-2025.pdf (accessed September 27, 2021).

Valente, T. W. 2012. Network interventions. *Science* 337(6090):49–53.

Valente, T. W., K. Fujimoto, C. P. Chou, and D. Spruijt-Metz. 2009. Adolescent affiliations and adiposity: A social network analysis of friendships and obesity. *The Journal of Adolescent Health* 45(2):202–204.

Vilela, S., M. M. Hetherington, A. Oliveira, and C. Lopes. 2018. Tracking diet variety in childhood and its association with eating behaviours related to appetite: The generation XXI birth cohort. *Appetite* 123:241–248.

Vilela, S., M. Severo, T. Moreira, A. Oliveira, M. M. Hetherington, and C. Lopes. 2019. Association between eating frequency and eating behaviours related to appetite from 4 to 7 years of age: Findings from the population-based birth cohort generation XXI. *Appetite* 132:82–90.

Wardle, J., C. A. Guthrie, S. Sanderson, and L. Rapoport. 2001. Development of the Children's Eating Behaviour Questionnaire. *Journal of Child Psychology and Psychiatry, and Allied Disciplines* 42(7):963–970.

Waters, H., and M. Graf. 2018. *America's obesity crisis: The health and economic costs of excess weight*. The Milken Institute. https://milkeninstitute.org/sites/default/files/reports-pdf/Mi-Americas-Obesity-Crisis-WEB.pdf (accessed October 11, 2021).

Weiss, D. J., A. Nelson, C. A. Vargas-Ruiz, K. Gligori , S. Bavadekar, E. Gabrilovich, A. Bertozzi-Villa, J. Rozier, H. S. Gibson, T. Shekel, C. Kamath, A. Lieber, K. Schulman, Y. Shao, V. Qarkaxhija, A. K. Nandi, S. H. Keddie, S. Rumisha, P. Amratia, R. Arambepola, et al. 2020. Global maps of travel time to healthcare facilities. *Nature Medicine* 26:1835–1838.

Woolf, S. H., D. A. Chapman, R. T. Sabo, and E. B. Zimmerman. 2021. Excess deaths from COVID-19 and other causes in the US, March 1, 2020, to January 2, 2021. *Journal of the American Medical Association* 325(17):1786–1789.

Zeevi, D., T. Korem, N. Zmora, D. Israeli, D. Rothschild, A. Weinberger, O. Ben-Yacov, D.Lador, T. Avnit-Sagi, M. Lotan-Pompan, J. Suez, J. A. Mahdi, E. Matot, G. Malka, N. Kosower, M. Rein, G. Zilberman-Schapira, L. Dohnalová, M. Pevsner-Fischer, R. Bikovsky, et al. 2015. Personalized nutrition by prediction of glycemic responses. *Cell* 163(5):P1079–1094.

Zhang, S., K. de la Haye, M. Ji, and R. An. 2018. Applications of social network analysis to obesity: A systematic review. *Obesity Reviews* 19(7):976–988.

Zhang, X., Q. Qi, C. Zhang, S. R. Smith, F. B. Hu, F. M. Sacks, G. A. Bray, and L. Qi. 2012. FTO genotype and 2-year change in body composition and fat distribution in response to weight-loss diets. *Diabetes* 61(11):3005–3011.

Appendix A

Workshop Agenda

Challenges and Opportunities for Precision and Personalized Nutrition

A Virtual Food Forum Workshop

August 10–12, 2021
All times in ET

10:00 AM   **Welcome & Opening Remarks**
Eric Decker, University of Massachusetts Amherst
Planning Committee Chair

SESSION 1: **The Current Evidence Base and Limitations**
Moderator: Cindy Davis, U.S. Department of Agriculture
Planning Committee Member

10:10   **Human Variability – A Basis for Precision and Personalized Nutrition**
John Mathers, Newcastle University

10:30   **Precision Nutrition at the Intersection of History and Genomics**
Constance Hilliard, University of North Texas

10:50   **Integrating Microbiome and Dietary Data**
             Abigail Johnson, University of Minnesota

11:10   **Opportunities and Obstacles in Precision Nutrition from an
             Engineering Perspective**
             Christian Metallo, Salk Institute

11:30   **Psychosocial Influences on Eating Behavior**
             Susan Carnell, The Johns Hopkins University

11:50   **Integration of Multiple Omics**
             Michael Snyder, Stanford University

12:10 PM   **Q&A and Panel Discussion**

1:00   **ADJOURN SESSION 1**

             SESSION 2 (August 11)

10:00 AM   **Summary of Day 1**
             *Cindy Davis, U.S. Department of Agriculture
             Planning Committee Member*

             SESSION 2: Innovative Methodologies and Technologies
             *Moderator: Bruce Y. Lee, CUNY Graduate School of Public
             Health & Health Policy
             Planning Committee Member*

10:15   **Industry Landscape in Personalized Nutrition**
             Mariëtte Abrahams, Qina

10:40   **The Genetic Scale**
             *Denise Ney, University of Wisconsin–Madison
             Jim Kaput, Vydiant
             Ahmed El-Sohemy, University of Toronto*

11:15   **The Physiology/Microbiome Scale**
             *Sarah Berry, King's College London
             Michal Rein, Weizmann Institute of Science
             Guru Banavar, Viome*

11:50   **The Individual Scale**
Andres Acosta, Mayo Clinic
Samantha Kleinberg, Stevens Institute of Technology
Diana M. Thomas, United States Military Academy at West Point

12:25 PM   **The Social-Ecological Scale**
Kayla de la Haye, University of Southern California
Sean Duffy, Omada Health
Michael Howell, Google Health

1:00   **ADJOURN SESSION 2**

SESSION 3 (August 12)

10:00 AM   **Summary of Day 1 and Day 2**
Bruce Y. Lee, CUNY Graduate School of Public Health &
Health Policy
Planning Committee Member

SESSION 3: **Implementation of Precision and Personalized Nutrition**
Moderator: Robin McKinnon, U.S. Food and Drug Administration
Planning Committee Member

10:15   **Will Precision Nutrition Help Us Achieve Greater Health Equity?**
Christina Roberto, University of Pennsylvania

10:30   **Challenges for Implementing Precision Nutrition**
Peter Lurie, Center for Science in the Public Interest

10:45   **Regulatory Perspective**
Rob Califf, Verily Life Science

11:00   **Commercializing Personal Nutrition**
Joshua Anthony, Nlumn

11:15   **Health Claims Communications to the Public**
Martin Hahn, Hogan Lovells

11:30   **Incorporating Precision Nutrition into Food-Based and Nutrient-Based Guidelines**
Patsy Brannon, Cornell University

11:45   **Q&A and Panel Discussion**

1:00 PM   **ADJOURN SESSION**

Appendix B

Acronyms and Abbreviations

AEBQ	Adult Eating Behavior Questionnaire
AI	artificial intelligence
ASN	American Society for Nutrition
BEBQ	Baby Eating Behavior Questionnaire
BEST	Biomarkers, EndpointS, and other Tools
BMI	body mass index
CDRR	chronic disease risk reduction
CEBQ	Child Eating Behavior Questionnaire
CFSAN	Center for Food Safety and Applied Nutrition
CLIA	Comprehensive Laboratory Improvement Act
CVD	cardiovascular disease
DIETFITS	Diet Intervention Examining the Factors Interacting with Treatment Success
DRI	Dietary Reference Intake
DSM-5	*Diagnostic and Statistical Manual of Mental Disorders, Fifth Edition*
EAR	estimated average requirement
FDA	U.S. Food and Drug Administration
FTC	Federal Trade Commission
FTO	fat mass and obesity-associated

GBD	global burden of disease
GRADE	Grading of Recommendations Assessment, Development and Evaluation
GWAS	genome-wide association studies
HHS	U.S. Department of Health and Human Services
INSNA	International Network of Social Network Analysis
LDL	low-density lipoprotein
LDT	laboratory-developed test
MacTel	macular telangiectasia
MS/MS	tandem mass spectrometry
NASEM	National Academy of Sciences, Engineering, and Medicine
NCI	National Cancer Institute
NHGRI	National Human Genome Research Institute
NHS	National Health Service
NIH	National Institutes of Health
ODS	Office of Dietary Supplements
PEACH lab	Psychology of Eating and Consumer Health laboratory
Phe	phenylalanine
PKU	phenylketonuria
PPGR	postprandial glucose response
PPT	personalized postprandial targeting
PREDICT	Personalized Responses to Dietary Composition Trial
PRS	polygenic risk score
RCT	randomized controlled trial
RDA	recommended dietary allowance
SNP	single nucleotide polymorphism
SPT	serine palmitoyl transferase
UL	tolerable upper level
UNC	University of North Carolina at Chapel Hill
USDA	U.S. Department of Agriculture
VLCADD	very-long-chain acyl-CoA dehydrogenase deficiency
WES	whole exome sequencing

Appendix C

Biographical Sketches of Workshop Speakers, Moderators, and Planning Committee Members

Mariëtte Abrahams, Ph.D., M.B.A., R.D., is founder and chief executive officer of Qina, a business-to-business platform and consultancy that provides access to a curated database of personalized nutrition solutions and a network of domain experts. She has been working in the clinical and medical nutrition industry for more than 20 years and leverages her combined expertise in nutrition, business, and research to help businesses navigate the personalized nutrition industry, provide market insights, and innovate. Dr. Abrahams received an M.B.A. from The Open University and a Ph.D. in personalized nutrition from the University of Bradford.

Andres J. Acosta, M.D., Ph.D., is a consultant in the Division of Gastroenterology and Hepatology, Department of Internal Medicine, at the Mayo Clinic, having joined the staff in 2016. He is also assistant professor of medicine in the Mayo Clinic College of Medicine and Science and provides mentorship to medical students, clinical fellows, and others. Dr. Acosta's main career goal is to understand and cure obesity. His research focuses on gastrointestinal physiology, utilizing a combination of genetics, physiology, pharmacology, proteomics, metabolomics, and gastrointestinal and brain imaging to understand food intake regulation and to modulate these factors for the treatment of obesity. He is principal investigator and coinvestigator on research funded by the National Institute of Diabetes and Digestive and Kidney Diseases. Dr. Acosta is a member of the American College of Gastroenterology, the American Gastroenterological Association, the American Society for Gastrointestinal Endoscopy, and The Obesity Society. He earned a B.S. in health science and an M.D. at Universidad San Francisco de Quito in Ecuador, graduating magna cum laude for both degrees. Dr. Acosta earned a Ph.D. in physiology and pharmacology at the University of Florida College of Medicine, and completed an internship and residency in internal medicine at the University of Florida Health Shands Hospital.

Joshua Anthony, Ph.D., M.B.A., M.S., is founder and chief executive officer at Nlumn, a consulting company that works with food, nutrition, and health-technology companies to help them compete in the personalized nutrition and health marketplace. Nlumn's mission is to make personalized nutrition accessible to help every individual make better choices and live a healthier life. Dr. Anthony has worked collaboratively to help launch more than 150 science-based nutrition products. Before starting Nlumn, he was founding chief science officer at the personalized nutrition company Habit. He was also vice president of global research and development in nutrition and health at the Campbell Soup Company. Prior to working with Habit and Campbell, Dr. Anthony held technical and management roles at Mead Johnson Nutrition and Unilever. He also served as an adjunct professor of physiology at the Indiana University School of Medicine. Dr. Anthony earned a B.S. in biological sciences from Carnegie Mellon University, an M.S. in nutritional sciences from the University of Illinois, an M.B.A. from Vanderbilt University, and a Ph.D. in cell and molecular physiology from the Pennsylvania State University College of Medicine.

Guruduth Banavar, Ph.D., M.B.A., M.S., is chief technology officer and leads the development of artificial intelligence (AI) systems at Viome, a company that offers unprecedented visibility into the human biological ecosystem and delivers personalized food and supplement recommendations to deter chronic disease. Until April 2017, he was a global vice president at IBM, leading Watson AI research. Dr. Banavar has built a range of advanced technologies and solutions in multiple industries throughout his career. He delivered the 2017 Turing Lecture, and has spoken at Nobel Prize award ceremonies, the Aspen Ideas Festival, and the Milken Conference. He received the Leadership in Technology Management Award from the Portland International Conference on Management of Engineering and Technology in 2017 and a National Innovation Award from the President of India in 2009. Dr. Banavar has served on New York Governor Andrew Cuomo's commission for state resiliency, and he was an elected member of the IBM Academy of Technology. He has published extensively and holds more than 30 U.S. patents. His work has been featured in international media outlets, including *The New York Times*, *The Economist*, *The Wall Street Journal*, the BBC, and NPR. Dr. Banavar holds a Ph.D. in computer science from the University of Utah.

Sarah Berry, Ph.D., M.Sc., is associate professor at King's College London and serves on the scientific advisory board for ZOE. Her research interests relate to the influence of dietary components on markers of cardiovascular disease risk, with a particular focus on precision nutrition, postprandial metabolism, and food and fat structure. Since commencing her research career at King's in 2000, Dr. Berry has been the academic leader for more than 30 human nutrition studies in cardiometabolic health. Ongoing research involves human and mechanistic studies to elucidate how markers of cardiometabolic health can be modulated following acute and chronic intakes of different fatty acids, as well as studies to investigate the influence of the food matrix on macro- and micronutrient release from different plant-based foods and subsequent effects on postprandial measures. Dr. Berry is also lead nutritional scientist on the PREDICT program, assessing the genetic, metabolic, metagenomic, and meal-dependent effects on metabolic responses to food in more than 6,000 individuals in the United Kingdom and United States. This research is at the forefront of developments in personalized nutrition and is forging a new way forward in the design and implementation of large-scale remote nutrition research studies integrating novel technologies, citizen science, and artificial intelligence. Dr. Berry is also academic lead on the COVID Symptom Study Diet and Lifestyle Questionnaire with 1.1 million participants, assessing diet and lifestyle behaviors before and during the COVID-19 pandemic and relationship with COVID-19 risk and obesity. She holds an M.Sc. and Ph.D. in nutrition from King's College London.

Patsy Brannon, Ph.D., R.D., is currently visiting professor, and was professor until her retirement in June 2018, in the Division of Nutritional Sciences at Cornell University, where she has also served as dean of the College of Human Ecology. Prior to moving to Cornell University, Dr. Brannon was chair of the Department of Nutrition and Food Science at the University of Maryland. She has also served as visiting professor at the Office of Dietary Supplements at the National Institutes of Health. Dr. Brannon's research focus includes nutritional and metabolic regulation of gene expression, especially relating to human development, the placenta, and exocrine pancreas. She was a member of the National Academies of Sciences, Engineering, and Medicine's committees on Dietary Reference Intakes for vitamin D and calcium and for sodium and potassium, as well as the National Academies' Food and Nutrition Board. Dr. Brannon was a member of a number of professional and scientific associations and has served on the executive board of the American Society for Nutrition (ASN). She has received numerous awards, including the ASN Fellow, Pew Faculty Scholar in Nutrition award, and the Centennial Laureate award from Florida State University. Dr. Brannon received her Ph.D. in nutritional biochemistry from Cornell University.

Robert (Rob) M. Califf, M.D., M.Acc, is head of clinical policy and strategy for Verily and Google Health. Prior to this, he was vice chancellor for health data science for the Duke University School of Medicine; director of Duke Forge, Duke's center for health data science; and the Donald F. Fortin, M.D., professor of cardiology. Dr. Califf served as deputy commissioner for medical products and tobacco in the U.S. Food and Drug Administration from 2015 to 2016, and as commissioner of food and drugs from 2016 to 2017. He was founding director of the Duke Clinical Research Institute and is one of the most frequently cited authors in biomedical science. A nationally and internationally recognized leader in cardiovascular medicine, health outcomes research, health care quality, and clinical research, Dr. Califf is a graduate of the Duke University School of Medicine.

Susan Carnell, Ph.D., is associate professor in the Division of Child and Adolescent Psychiatry, Department of Psychiatry and Behavioral Sciences, at Johns Hopkins University School of Medicine, where she heads the Appetite Lab. A central question motivating her research is, "Why do some people develop obesity while others do not?" Dr. Carnell's research program investigates the model that individuals differ in appetite-related biobehavioral traits (e.g., food cue responsiveness, satiety sensitivity) that manifest early in life, show genetic influence, and interact with environmental factors to predict eating behaviors and weight trajectories. To probe this model she employs a range of methods including behavioral tests, questionnaires, genotyping, hormonal assays, and neuroimaging techniques. Ongoing research projects include investigations of appetite and body weight in infants, children, adolescents, and adults, including studies of bariatric surgery and eating disorders. Dr. Carnell received a B.A. in experimental psychology from the University of Oxford and a Ph.D. in health psychology at University College London, and she completed postdoctoral training at Columbia University.

Cindy D. Davis, Ph.D., serves as national program leader for the Human Nutrition Program conducted by the U.S. Department of Agricultural (USDA) Agricultural Research Service. In this role, she helps direct the scientific program for six Human Nutrition Research Centers. Prior to joining USDA, Dr. Davis was director of grants and extramural activities in the Office of Dietary Supplements (ODS), where she actively engaged and encouraged partnerships with other National Institutes of Health (NIH) institutes and centers to develop a portfolio for advancing both nutritional and botanical dietary supplement research for optimizing public health. She is actively involved in a number of government working groups focused on the microbiome, including as cofounder and cochair of the Joint Agency Microbiome (NIH, Food and Drug Administration, National Institute of

Standards and Technology, and USDA) working group. Before coming to ODS, Dr. Davis was a program director in the Nutritional Sciences Research Group at the National Cancer Institute. She completed her post-doctoral training at the Laboratory of Experimental Carcinogenesis at the National Cancer Institute, and then joined the Grand Forks Human Nutrition Research Center, USDA, as a research nutritionist. In 2000, Dr. Davis received a Presidential Early Career Award for Scientists and Engineers and was named the USDA Early Career Scientist. She has published more than 135 peer-reviewed journal articles and 11 invited book chapters, and she is a supplement editor for the *Journal of Nutrition*, assistant editor for *Nutrition Reviews*, and a member of the editorial board for *Advances in Nutrition*. Dr. Davis received a B.S. degree in nutritional sciences with honors from Cornell University and a Ph.D. degree in nutrition with a minor in human cancer biology from the University of Wisconsin–Madison.

Eric A. Decker, Ph.D., M.S., is professor and head of the Department of Food Science at the University of Massachusetts Amherst (UMass), and has served since 2008 as director of the UMass Food Science Industry Strategic Research Alliance. Dr. Decker is actively conducting research to characterize mechanisms of lipid oxidation, antioxidant protection of foods, and the health implications of bioactive lipids. He has authored more than 430 publications and has been listed as one of the most highly cited scientists in agriculture since 2005. Dr. Decker has served on numerous committees for such institutions as the Food and Drug Administration; the National Academies of Sciences, Engineering, and Medicine; the Institute of Food Technologists; the U.S. Department of Agriculture; and the American Heart Association. He has received recognition for his research and service from the American Oil Chemist Society, the Agriculture and Food Chemistry Division of the American Chemical Society, the Institute of Food Technologists, UMass, and the University of Kentucky. Dr. Decker has also been elected to serve as an officer for the American Meat Science Association and the Institute of Food Technologists, and, most recently, as the president of the American Oil Chemist Society. He holds an M.S. in food science and nutrition from Washington State University and a Ph.D. in food science and nutrition from the University of Massachusetts Amherst.

Kayla de la Haye, Ph.D., is associate professor of population and public health sciences at the University of Southern California. She works to address key public health issues by integrating behavioral science, network science, and systems science, focusing on family and community social networks and the environments in which people live, to promote healthy eating and food security and to prevent diet-related diseases and health disparities. Her research also explores the role of social networks in how families, teams, and coalitions solve complex problems and address health risks. Previously, Dr. de la Haye worked as an associate behavioral/social scientist at the RAND Corporation. She serves on the executive committee of the International Network of Social Network Analysis (INSNA), and in 2018, she received the INSNA Freeman Award for significant contributions to the study of social structure. Dr. de la Haye holds a Ph.D. in psychology from the University of Adelaide in Australia.

Sean Duffy is cofounder and chief executive officer of Omada Health, a digital care program that empowers people to achieve their health goals through sustainable lifestyle change. In 2017, Omada was recognized as one of Fast Company's Most Innovative Companies, and in 2016, the company was named a Technology Pioneer by the World Economic Forum. Prior to Omada, he worked at both Google and IDEO. Recognized as a thought leader on the future of health care, Mr. Duffy has written or spoken extensively in *The New England Journal of Medicine* and *The Wall Street Journal*, and at the World Economic Forum. A former M.D./M.B.A. candidate at Harvard, he holds a B.S. in neuroscience from Columbia University.

Ahmed El-Sohemy, Ph.D., is professor and Canada research chair in nutrigenomics at the University of Toronto. He joined the faculty in 2000 to establish a research program in nutrigenomics, with the goal of identifying biomarkers of dietary exposure and elucidating the genetic basis for variability in nutrient response and dietary preferences. Dr. El-Sohemy collaborates with researchers across Canada, as well as the United States, Costa Rica, Denmark, Italy, Switzerland, South Korea, and Singapore. He has published more than 70 peer-reviewed articles and has given almost 100 invited talks around the world. Dr. El-Sohemy is on the editorial board of eight journals and served as an expert reviewer for more than 30 scientific and medical journals and 12 granting agencies. He earned a Ph.D. in nutritional sciences from the University of Toronto and completed a postdoctoral fellowship at the Harvard T.H. Chan School of Public Health.

Martin Hahn, J.D., is partner at Hogan Lovells, where he uses his background in food technology and his comprehensive understanding of the laws governing the food industry to help clients navigate through the countless regulatory and business issues impacting the industry from farm to table. He recognizes the demands clients face and finds innovative and creative solutions, particularly when responding to observations raised by regulators during inspections. Mr. Hahn has handled almost every issue impacting the food industry and has developed a comprehensive understanding of the laws affecting the labeling and advertising of foods, dietary supplements, infant formulas, medical foods, foods for special dietary use, and hemp extracts when positioned as a food or dietary supplement. He helps anticipate new trends and develops the data needed to distinguish a client's products from others on the market. Mr. Hahn uses his understanding of science and technology in the food industry to provide assistance in obtaining regulatory authorizations to market new food ingredients, food packaging materials, and dietary ingredients. He holds a J.D. from Northwestern University.

Constance Hilliard, Ph.D., M.A., is professor of evolutionary history at the University of North Texas. In recent years, she has pioneered the field of African evolutionary history, a discipline emerging at the intersection of environmental history and genomics, offering previously overlooked clues as to the etiology of certain health disparities for which Americans of African descent have unusually high susceptibilities. Her Ancestral Gene Variants Model identifies certain beneficial ancestral gene variants in the unique ecology of the West Africa interior, which may become maladaptive in the U.S. dietary culture, particularly as relates to calcium and sodium intake. Dr. Hilliard received a B.A., M.A., and Ph.D. in history from Harvard University.

Michael Howell, M.D., M.P.H., is chief clinical officer and deputy chief health officer at Google, where he focuses on how technology can help improve health and health care. He was previously chief quality officer at the University of Chicago Medicine, where he was the senior physician responsible for overseeing the quality of care at the health system. Before that, Dr. Howell served at Harvard Medical School and the Beth Israel Deaconess Medical Center in a variety of roles focused on quality, patient safety, and health care delivery science. An active investigator, he has published more than 100 research articles, editorials, and book chapters. These studies have been covered by CNN, *The New York Times, The Wall Street Journal, Forbes,* and *Consumer Reports,* among others. A nationally recognized expert on patient safety and quality, Dr. Howell has also served on national advisory and guideline panels for the Centers for Disease Control and Prevention, Medicare, the National Academy of Medicine, and national professional associations. His book, *Understanding Healthcare Delivery Science,* focuses on the intersection of real-world improvement and research quality methods in the complex environment of health care. He holds an M.P.H. and M.D. from Harvard University.

Abigail (Abby) Johnson, Ph.D., R.D., is assistant professor and registered dietitian in the Division of Epidemiology and Community Health in the School of Public Health at the University of Minnesota. She is also associate director of the Nutrition Coordinating Center, which distributes and supports the Nutrition Data System for Research. Dr. Johnson has diverse experiences in nutrition research, ranging from molecular biology and clinical nutrition to bioinformatics and public health. Her present research explores the relationships between diet and the human gut microbiome in health and disease using novel computational methods to integrate dietary data with other multiomics data. She has demonstrated that daily changes in dietary intake and overall dietary patterns are reflected in shifts in microbial composition in humans. Dr. Johnson received a B.S. in nutrition and biology and a Ph.D. in nutrition from the University of Minnesota. Her training has included industry postdoctoral work with Nestle Health Science and academic postdoctoral training in bioinformatics and the microbiome under the mentorship of Dr. Dan Knights at the University of Minnesota.

Jim Kaput, Ph.D., is cofounder and chief scientific officer of Vydiant, which is developing a comprehensive knowledge base of factors affecting health and disease, using digital health tools to deliver personalized recommendations to individuals. He has been developing strategies and methods to target nutrition for improving personal and public health for his entire career. Dr. Kaput was a staff and biochemistry faculty member at the University of Illinois College of Medicine, director of the Northwestern University Biotechnology Laboratory, and coordinator of science and administrative activities for the National Center for Minority Health and Health Disparities Center of Excellence in Nutritional Genomics at the University of California, Davis. From 2007 to 2011, he was director of the Division of Personalized Nutrition and Medicine at the U.S. Food and Drug Administration's National Center for Toxicological Research, where his team collaborated with the U.S. Department of Agriculture and the Boys, Girls, Adults Community Development Center in Marvell, Arkansas. Dr. Kaput was a member of the executive committee of NuGO (Nutrigenomics Organization) for 8 years, and for 5 years he was coeditor of *Genes & Nutrition*. His most recent past position was senior expert at the Nestle Institute of Health Sciences from 2011 to 2017. Dr. Kaput received a Ph.D. from Colorado State University in biochemistry and molecular biology and spent 5 years as a postdoctoral fellow and assistant professor at the Rockefeller University in the laboratory of Günter Blobel, the 1999 Nobel laureate in physiology and medicine.

Samantha Kleinberg, Ph.D., is associate professor of computer science at Stevens Institute of Technology. She received the National Science Foundation's CAREER award and the Complex Systems Scholar award from the James S. McDonnell Foundation, and she is a 2016 Kavli fellow of the National Academy of Sciences. Dr. Kleinberg is author of *Causality,*

Probability, and Time (Cambridge University Press, 2012) and *Why: A Guide to Finding and Using Causes* (O'Reilly Media, 2015), and she is editor of *Time and Causality Across the Sciences* (Cambridge University Press, 2019). She received a Ph.D. in computer science from New York University and was a computing innovation fellow at Columbia University in the Department of Biomedical Informatics.

Katie Koecher, Ph.D., is associate expert nutrition scientist at General Mills Bell Institute of Health and Nutrition, where she leads the nutrition research strategic plan and pipeline development and conducts research on carbohydrates and health, weight management, diabetes, and, more recently, personalized nutrition. She has held various positions in food science and nutrition, including product developer at Nestle Health Science and contract microbiologist for 3M. Currently, Dr. Koecher serves as committee cochair for the Institute for the Advancement of Food and Nutrition Sciences (previously ILSI-North America) carbohydrate committee. She completed a Ph.D. in food science and nutrition at the University of Minnesota.

Bruce Y. Lee, M.D., M.B.A., is professor of health policy and management at the City University of New York Graduate School of Public Health & Health Policy, where he is executive director of Public Health Computational and Operations Research and executive director of the Center for Advanced Technology and Communication in Health. He is a systems modeler, and a computational and digital health expert, writer, and health journalist. Dr. Lee has more than two decades' experience in industry and academia, developing mathematical and computational models to assist a wide range of decision makers in health and public health. Dr. Lee is a senior contributor for *Forbes*, covering a wide range of health-related topics, and his writing has also appeared in other media outlets, including *The New York Times*, *Time*, *The Guardian*, *HuffPost*, and *MIT Technology Review*. He holds an M.B.A. from Stanford Graduate School of Business and an M.D. from Harvard Medical School.

Peter Lurie, M.D., M.P.H., is president of the Center for Science in the Public Interest. Previously, he was associate commissioner for public health strategy and analysis at the Food and Drug Administration, where he worked on antimicrobial resistance, transparency, caffeinated beverages, arsenic in rice, fish consumption by pregnant and nursing women, expanded access to investigational drugs, and prescription drug abuse. Prior to that, Dr. Lurie was deputy director of Public Citizen's Health Research Group, where he addressed drug and device issues, coauthored the organization's *Worst Pills, Best Pills* consumer guide to medications, and led efforts to reduce worker exposure to hexavalent chromium and beryllium.

Earlier, as a faculty member at the University of California, San Francisco, and the University of Michigan, he studied needle exchange programs, ethical aspects of mother-to-infant HIV transmission studies, and other HIV policy issues domestically and abroad. Dr. Lurie earned an M.D. from the Albert Einstein College of Medicine.

John Mathers, Ph.D., is professor of human nutrition, director of the Human Nutrition Research Centre, and director of the Centre for Healthier Lives in Newcastle University in the United Kingdom. His major research interests are in understanding how eating patterns influence risks of age-related diseases, including heart disease, diabetes, dementia, and bowel cancer, using genomic and epigenomics approaches to understand the mechanisms though which nutrition influences cell function and, ultimately, health. Dr. Mathers led the European Union–funded Food4Me intervention study, which used a web-based approach to deliver a personalized nutrition intervention across seven European countries. He has a long-term interest in developing and implementing large-scale human intervention studies to improve healthy aging, and to reduce the risk of common age-related diseases, including bowel cancer and dementia. Dr. Mathers is past president of the Nutrition Society and has served on numerous grants panels and other committees for the Medical Research Council, Biotechnology and Biological Sciences Research Council, Economic and Social Research Council, World Cancer Research Fund, and other research funders. He is a trustee of the British Nutrition Foundation and of the Rank Prize Funds, and is editor-in-chief of the *British Journal of Nutrition*. Dr. Mathers was an undergraduate in Newcastle and undertook his Ph.D. and postdoctoral research in the University of Cambridge, followed by a research fellow post in Edinburgh University before being appointed in Newcastle.

Josiemer Mattei, Ph.D., M.S., M.P.H., is Donald and Sue Pritzker associate professor of nutrition at the Department of Nutrition at Harvard T.H. Chan School of Public Health. She investigates genetic, dietary, and psychosocial determinants of cardiometabolic diseases in racial and ethnic groups and underserved populations, as a framework to explain health disparities, using observational studies and culturally tailored community interventions. Dr. Mattei recently served as a panelist for the National Institutes of Health workshop on Precision Nutrition: Research Gaps and Opportunities, presenting on social determinants of health and inequities in precision nutrition. She is a Robert Wood Johnson Foundation Culture of Health Leader and received the Mark Bieber Award for Outstanding Nutrition-related Research by the American Heart Association. Dr. Mattei obtained an M.P.H. in epidemiology and biostatistics and a Ph.D. in nutritional biochemistry from Tufts University.

Robin McKinnon, Ph.D., M.P.A., is senior advisor for nutrition policy at the Food and Drug Administration (FDA) Center for Food Safety and Applied Nutrition (CFSAN), where she works to advance nutrition-related activities across CFSAN, including FDA's Nutrition Innovation Strategy. Prior to joining FDA, she was a health policy specialist at the National Cancer Institute (NCI) of the National Institutes of Health. At NCI, Dr. McKinnon led policy-relevant research initiatives on diet, obesity, and physical activity. She previously served on the planning committee for the 2009 National Academies of Sciences, Engineering, and Medicine workshop on The Public Health Effects of Food Deserts. Dr. McKinnon earned an M.P.A. from Harvard University and a Ph.D. in public policy and administration from George Washington University.

Christian Metallo, Ph.D., M.S., is professor at the Salk Institute for Biological Studies and adjunct professor of bioengineering at the University of California, San Diego. He studies how diet, genetics, and other factors alter metabolism to drive such diseases as cancer and neuropathy. Dr. Metallo's work focuses on mapping the biochemical networks sustaining biosynthesis and bioenergetics to uncover the mechanistic basis of disease and identify new therapeutic strategies. Using stable isotope tracers and advanced mass spectroscopy techniques, his lab quantifies how metabolic pathways are altered in cells, animal models, and patients. Taking this approach, Dr. Metallo has made key discoveries about the metabolic pathways that drive cancer progression and macular disease—pathways that can be influenced through dietary manipulations or targeted therapies. He was recently elected a fellow of the American Institute for Medical and Biological Engineering. Dr. Metallo received a B.S. in chemical engineering from the University of Pennsylvania and an M.S. and Ph.D. in chemical and biological engineering from the University of Wisconsin–Madison. He was a postdoctoral fellow at the Massachusetts Institute of Technology.

Denise M. Ney, Ph.D., R.D.N., is professor in the Department of Nutritional Sciences at the University of Wisconsin–Madison, where she served as department chair and director of the Interdepartmental Graduate Program in Nutritional Sciences. For more than 25 years, she has conducted research on how nutrition impacts gastrointestinal physiology and rare genetic diseases, focusing on the neuroendocrine regulation of intestinal adaptation and phenylketonuria (PKU), an inherited metabolic disorder that requires lifelong dietary restriction of the amino acid phenylalanine (Phe) to prevent cognitive impairment. Dr. Ney invented a way to use glycomacropeptide, a whey protein produced during cheesemaking, to formulate low-Phe medical foods, resulting in improved health for individuals with PKU worldwide. For this research, she is recognized as a Rare Disease Hero by the Food and Drug Administration's Office of Orphan Products Development, and is the recipient of the Spitze Land Grant Faculty Award from the College of Agriculture and Life Sciences and the Mary Schwartz Rose and Fellow awards from the American Society for Nutrition. Dr. Ney has mentored 13 Ph.D. students within her research program, many of whom hold faculty positions, and she directed the Didactic Program in Dietetics leading to more than 1,000 students achieving careers as registered dietitian nutritionists. She has published 135 research articles and 10 book chapters and is an inventor on two patents. Dr. Ney received a Ph.D. in nutrition science from the University of California, Davis.

Michal Rein, M.Sc., R.D., is pursuing a Ph.D. under joint supervision of Eran Segal from the Weizmann Institute of Science and Shira Zelber-Sagi from the University of Haifa. She is a registered dietitian, specializing in dietary interventions and modifications, and leads studies observing the effect of personally tailored diets by predictions of glycemic responses aimed to improve glycemic status and other metabolic parameters in various populations (such as healthy individuals, subjects with glucose intolerance, and breast cancer survivors). Additionally, Ms. Rein is a part of ongoing research integrating the data of dietary intake, personal characteristics, microbiome features and omics data on the influences of the individual reaction to glucose and other health indicators.

Christina A. Roberto, Ph.D., is Mitchell J. Blutt and Margo Krody Blutt presidential associate professor of health policy at the Perelman School of Medicine at the University of Pennsylvania (Penn). She is also director of the Psychology of Eating and Consumer Health laboratory (PEACH lab) and associate director of the Center for Health Incentives and Behavioral Economics at Penn. The mission of the PEACH lab is to identify and evaluate policies and interventions that promote healthy eating habits and prevent nutrition-related chronic diseases. The lab strives to help create a just and equitable food system in which those with the fewest resources and opportunities have the same chance to live a long, healthy life as those with the most. The PEACH lab works closely with policy makers and influencers to ask important, creative, and timely research questions that provide policy makers and institutions with science-based guidance. Dr. Roberto has an undergraduate degree in psychology from Princeton University, where she graduated magna cum laude; she earned a joint Ph.D. in clinical psychology and chronic disease epidemiology at Yale University. Additionally, Dr. Roberto completed a clinical internship at the Yale School of Medicine and was a Robert Wood Johnson Foundation health and society scholar at the Harvard T.H. Chan School of Public Health.

Nicholas J. Schork, Ph.D., M.A., is deputy director and distinguished professor of quantitative medicine at the Translational Genomics Research Institute. He is also adjunct professor of population sciences and molecular and cellular biology at City of Hope, adjunct professor of psychiatry and biostatistics at the University of California, San Diego, and adjunct professor of integrative structural and computational biology at the Scripps Research Institute. Prior to his current positions, Dr. Schork was professor and director of human biology at the J. Craig Venter Institute, professor of molecular and experimental medicine at Scripps Research, and director of bioinformatics and biostatistics for the Scripps Translational Science Institute. Between 1999 and 2000, he took a leave of absence from Case Western Reserve University to conduct research as vice president of statistical genomics at the French biotechnology company Genset, where he helped guide efforts to construct the first high-density map of genetic variation in the human genome. He has published more than 550 articles in many areas of biomedical and translation science, as well as areas of integrated nutrigenomics and the design of personalized nutritional trials. He was a member of the National Academies of Sciences, Engineering, and Medicine's Food and Nutrition Board from 2003 to 2007, and has a long history of collaborative and consortium-related research, in which he has contributed analysis methodology and applied data analysis expertise. Dr. Schork has 12 patents associated with genetic analysis methodology, has been involved with more than 10 start-up companies, and has mentored more than 75 students and postdoctoral fellows. He earned a Ph.D. in genetic epidemiology from the University of Michigan.

Michael Snyder, Ph.D., is Stanford Ascherman professor and chair of genetics and director of the Center of Genomics and Personalized Medicine at Stanford University. He is a leader in functional genomics and multiomics and is one of the major participants of the Encyclopedia of DNA Elements project. His laboratory was the first to perform a large-scale functional genomics project in any organism and has developed many technologies in genomics and proteomics, developing technologies for characterizing genomes, proteomes, and regulatory networks. Seminal findings from the Snyder Laboratory include the discovery that much more of the human genome is transcribed and contains regulatory information than was previously appreciated, and that a high diversity of transcription factor binding occurs both between and within species. Dr. Snyder launched the field of personalized medicine by combining different state-of-the-art omics technologies to perform the first longitudinal detailed integrative personal omics profile of a person, and his laboratory pioneered the use of wearable technologies (smart watches and continuous glucose monitoring) for precision health. He is cofounder of many biotechnology companies, including Personalis, SensOmics, Qbio, January, Protos, Oralome, Mirvie, and Filtricine. Dr. Snyder received Ph.D. training at the California Institute of Technology and carried out postdoctoral training at Stanford University.

Patrick J. Stover, Ph.D., is vice chancellor and dean for agriculture and life sciences at Texas A&M AgriLife, and director of Texas A&M AgriLife Research. As vice chancellor, he oversees coordination and collaboration of the agriculture, academic, and research programs across the Texas A&M University System, as well as four state agencies: Texas A&M AgriLife Research, Texas A&M AgriLife Extension Service, Texas A&M Veterinary Medical Diagnostic Laboratory, and Texas A&M Forest Service. Dr. Stover is also director of AgriLife Research, where he oversees 13 research centers across the state with a research portfolio of more than 500 projects and $214.2 million in annual research funding. As dean of the College of Agriculture and Life Sciences, Dr. Stover leads more than 7,000 students and 330 faculty members in 15 academic departments. He previously directed the Division of Nutritional Sciences at Cornell University. An international leader in biochemistry and nutrition, Dr. Stover focuses his research on the biochemical, genetic, and epigenetic mechanisms that underlie the relationships between folic acid and human pathologies, such as developmental anomalies, neuropathies, and cancer. He is an elected member of the National Academy of Sciences and a fellow of the American Association for the Advancement of Science. He is also former president of the American Society for Nutrition and has served two terms on the National Academies of Sciences, Engineering, and Medicine's Food and Nutrition Board. Dr. Stover received a Ph.D. in biochemistry and molecular biophysics from the Medical College of Virginia.

Diana M. Thomas, Ph.D., is professor of mathematical sciences at the United States Military Academy at West Point. She has been an active research mathematician for more than 25 years, with a focus on nutrition and obesity-related modeling, working with large, complex, and high-dimensional datasets. Dr. Thomas coinvented the remote weight loss program, SmartLoss™, which has been clinically applied worldwide to guide and improve individual patient weight loss adherence through smartphone technology. She has published more than 150 peer-reviewed articles and has led the development of more than 10 freely accessible health calculators. Dr. Thomas is associate editor of the *American Journal of Clinical Nutrition* and coedits the series "Best (but oft-forgotten) practices," consisting of methodologic commentaries or statistical tutorials, and also serves as editor for *Nutrition and Diabetes* and the *European Journal of Clinical Nutrition*. She has held governance positions in The Obesity Society, the American

Society of Nutrition, and the Mathematical Association of America. Dr. Thomas holds the 2012 Mathematical Association of America New Jersey Section Distinguished Teaching Award and the 2015 Obesity Society George Bray Founder's Award. She received a Ph.D. from the Georgia Institute of Technology and completed a National Research Council–funded postdoctoral fellowship at the United States Military Academy and the Army Research Laboratory.

Steven Zeisel, M.D., Ph.D., is Kenan distinguished university professor in nutrition and pediatrics, director of the Nutrition Research Institute, and director of the University of North Carolina at Chapel Hill (UNC) Nutrition Obesity Research Center, as well as founder and scientific advisor for SNP Therapeutics. The Nutrition Research Institute focuses on using genetic, epigenetic, and metabolomic methods to discover why there is individual variation in responses to and requirements for nutrients. The UNC Nutrition Obesity Research Center is one of 12 centers of excellence in nutrition research funded by the National Institutes of Health. Dr. Zeisel's research focuses on dietary requirements for the nutrient choline, genetic variation as a source of individual differences in requirements for and responses to nutrients, effects of choline and folate on stem cell proliferation, and apoptosis and resulting effects on health. SNP Therapeutics develops tests to detect gene variants that alter the metabolism of nutrients and result in health problems. Dr. Zeisel has authored more than 300 peer-reviewed scientific papers. He holds an M.D. from Harvard Medical School and a Ph.D. in nutrition from Massachusetts Institute of Technology.